AIDS Policy in Uganda

AIDS Policy in Uganda

Evidence, Ideology, and the Making of an African Success Story

John Kinsman

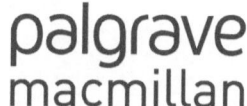

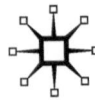

First published in 2010 by
PALGRAVE MACMILLAN®
in the United States – a division of St. Martin's Press
LLC, 175 Fifth Avenue, New York, NY 10010.

Where this book is distributed in the UK, Europe and the rest of the world,
this is by Palgrave Macmillan, a division of Macmillan Publishers Limited,
registered in England, company number 785998, of Houndmills, Basingstoke,
Hampshire RG21 6XS.

Palgrave Macmillan is the global academic imprint of the above companies
and has companies and representatives throughout the world.

Palgrave® and Macmillan® are registered trademarks in the United States, the
United Kingdom, Europe and other countries.

ISBN: 978–0–230–10428–0

Library of Congress Cataloging-in-Publication Data

Kinsman, John, 1964–
    AIDS policy in Uganda : evidence, ideology, and the making of an
African success story / John Kinsman.
        p. ; cm.
    Includes bibliographical references.
    ISBN 978-0-230-10428-0 (alk. paper)
    1. AIDS (Disease)—Uganda.   I. Title.
    [DNLM: 1. Acquired Immunodeficiency Syndrome—prevention &
control—Uganda. 2. Communicable Disease Control—history—Uganda.
3. HIV Infections—prevention & control—Uganda. 4. Health Policy—
history—Uganda. 5. History, 20th Century—Uganda. 6. History,
21st Century—Uganda. WC 503.6 K56a 2010]
    RA643.86.U33K56 2010
    362.196'97920096761—dc22

                                                                    2010000108

A catalogue record of the book is available from the British Library.

Design by MPS Limited, A Macmillan Company

First edition: August 2010

10 9 8 7 6 5 4 3 2 1

For Sabina

Contents

Figures and Tables

Acknowledgments

I needed a nudge of encouragement to write this book, and I received this nudge late in the year 2000, over an evening drink in Entebbe with my friend and colleague, Robert Pool. He suggested I approach the Amsterdam School for Social science Research (ASSR) to pursue a PhD that would investigate some of the questions that had arisen in my mind during five years with the Medical Research Council Programme on AIDS in Uganda. He had written his own PhD at the ASSR several years earlier, and he recommended that I contact Sjaak van der Geest to ask if he would agree to act as my supervisor for the doctoral thesis that eventually turned into this book. The project would never even have reached the starting blocks if Robert had not given me this introduction, and if Sjaak had not accepted to take me on.

When I moved to Amsterdam, in 2003, I was given an unprecedented level of trust and freedom to pursue my ideas. But I also received invaluable intellectual input from Sjaak and my PhD co-supervisor, Anita Hardon, and I thank them for the expert and invariably sound guidance that they provided throughout the process. I have learned a great deal from them both.

The ASSR itself offered extremely generous financial support for me to conduct my multisited fieldwork, and for that I am very grateful. My colleagues at the School also contributed greatly to my work through their constructively critical comments. I thank in particular Ellen Blommaert, Christine Dedding, Lotte Hoek, Marie Lindegaard, Eileen Moyer, Rachel Spronk, and Getnet Tadele. Special appreciation is due to Joost Beuving, Trudie Gerrits, and Josien de Klerk, both for their exceptional friendships and for the time and energy they expended reading and commenting on chapter drafts.

It goes without saying that this book could never have been written without the cooperation of my respondents. All of them took valuable and sometimes quite extended periods from their work—in the office, in the clinic, or in the fields—to talk with me, and I extend to them all my deepest gratitude. I have tried my utmost to remain faithful to the spirit and the letter of what they told me, and I sincerely hope I have managed to do so.

I am especially grateful to the following people for their particular contributions to my fieldwork: Edward Kirumira in Kampala, who provided essential support to my request for official clearance to conduct fieldwork in Uganda; Julius Ecuru of the Uganda National Council for Science and Technology, who provided that clearance; Ned Kanyesigye, my former, and extremely well-connected, colleague from Masaka, who was very generous in supplying me with the names and contact details of potential respondents; Ssalongo Mugerwa in Masaka, who proved to be not only a safe and reliable driver on Uganda's treacherous roads but also excellent company on the many bumpy journeys that we shared into the hinterland; and Brent Wolff, who, with his family, took over Sabina's and my house and dog when we left Masaka in 2001, and who welcomed me back upon my return with delicious meals and all-important updates on developments in the district.

My children Pascal and Amanda both appeared during the period in which I was writing the book, and it would be fair to say that they were not especially helpful in the process. So I can't thank them for that, but I can thank them for being the most beautiful additions to my life that I could ever have dreamed of. This brings me, naturally, to Sabina, my wife and first-line editorial critic. Thank you for your endless support throughout this long and winding road. I couldn't have traveled it without you.

Permissions

Cover artwork courtesy of Margaret Nagawa

Map of Uganda and neighboring countries created by Magnus Strömgren, partly based on GIS data from ESRI.

Permission to quote the December 1984 *Star* article, entitled "Mysterious Disease kills 100 people in Rakai" was granted by Drake Sekeba.

Wilson Carswell granted permission to quote from his unpublished memoirs.

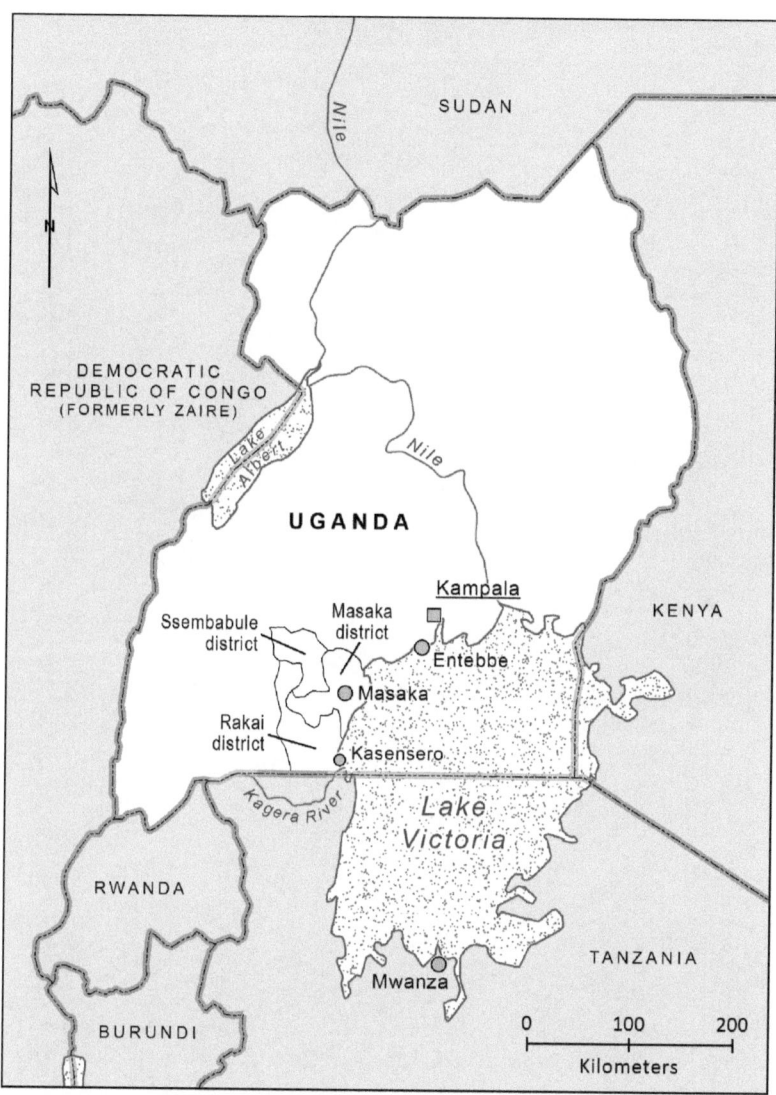

Uganda and neighboring countries.

Acronyms and Abbreviations

ABC	Abstain, Be faithful, or use a Condom
ACP	AIDS Control Programme (Uganda)
AHF	AIDS Healthcare Foundation (USA)
AIDS	Acquired Immunodeficiency Syndrome
APC	AIDS Prevention Committee
ART	Antiretroviral therapy
ARV	Antiretroviral drug
AZT	Azidothymidine (more commonly known as Zidovudine)
DAI	Drug Access Initiative
DHS	Demographic and Health Surveys
DSSC	Disease Surveillance Sub-Committee
EBM	Evidence-Based Medicine
EBP	Evidence-Based Policy
GFATM	Global Fund to Fight AIDS, Tuberculosis and Malaria
HAART	Highly Active Antiretroviral Therapy (also known as Triple Therapy)
HIV	Human Immunodeficiency Virus
HTLV-III	Human T-lymphotropic Virus type III
IEC	Information, Education and Communication
JCRC	Joint Clinical Research Centre (Uganda)
KAP	Knowledge, Attitude, and Practice
KS	Kaposi's Sarcoma
LAV	Lymphadenopathy Associated Virus
MDG	Millennium Development Goal
MIT	Masaka Intervention Trial (Uganda)

MoH	Ministry of Health (Uganda)
MRC	Medical Research Council Programme on AIDS in Uganda
MSF	Médecins Sans Frontières
NDA	National Drug Authority (Uganda)
NGO	Non-Governmental Organization
ODI	Overseas Development Institute
OI	Opportunistic Infection
OR	Operational Research
PC	Parish Coordinator
PEPFAR	The U.S. President's Emergency Plan for AIDS Relief
PHC	Primary Health Care
PHLS	Public Health Laboratory Service (England)
PMTCT	Prevention of Mother-to-Child Transmission (of HIV)
RC	Resistance Council
RCT	Randomized Controlled Trial
STD	Sexually Transmitted Disease
STI	Sexually Transmitted Infection
TASO	The AIDS Support Organisation (Uganda)
TB	Tuberculosis
TPDF	Tanzanian People's Defence Forces
UAC	Uganda AIDS Commission
UNAIDS	United Nations Joint Programme on HIV/AIDS
USAID	United States Agency for International Development
UVRI	Uganda Virus Research Institute
VCT	Voluntary Counseling and Testing (for HIV)
WHO	World Health Organization
'3 by 5'	WHO-driven plan for global ARV scale-up. The idea was to have 3 million people with AIDS receiving ART by the end of the year 2005.

I

Introduction

A Call to Arms

The grey-haired old man had to be helped up the steps onto the stage, and he walked slowly over to his chair, beaming at the warm reception and applause that he was receiving. He sat for a moment and listened as the conference chairman introduced him, describing him as "an icon of our times"; and then he stood to address the 12,000 delegates attending the closing ceremony of the Thirteenth International AIDS Conference.

Held in July 2000 in Durban, South Africa—then the country with more HIV-positive people than any other in the world—this conference had been beset by controversy even before it started. The meeting's slogan was "Break the Silence," and silence was indeed in short supply. Disputes were raging in South Africa over the cause of AIDS, with different groups pointing to HIV, to poverty-induced malnutrition, or even to the antiretroviral drugs used to treat the condition (*New York Times*, 2000; *Sunday Independent*, 2000). The protagonists on all sides held deeply entrenched views, with the mainstream scientific community holding firmly to the position that HIV causes AIDS (Durban Declaration, 2000), and South African President Thabo Mbeki allying himself with the so-called AIDS dissidents who believed in the various alternatives (Epstein, 2007: 106–108). It was a classic case of the complex interplay between politics and science, and it had been the focus of much anger and angst during the conference.

But now, Nelson Mandela saw the opportunity to put the discussion back—as he saw it—on track. His speech to the conference was carefully crafted, and it touched on several important themes. Mention was made of the controversy in South Africa, but in what some saw as a reprimand to his successor, the former President argued that this acrimonious debate should now be consigned to history. The urgency of the situation demanded that attention be turned fully to reversing the inadequate response that had prevailed across most of the African continent since the very first AIDS cases were identified around the border between Uganda and Tanzania way back in the early 1980s.

"The ordinary people of this continent," he pointed out with an unmatched authority, "and of the world—and particularly the poor who on our continent will again carry a disproportionate burden of this scourge—would, if anyone cared to ask their opinions, wish that the dispute about the primacy of politics or science be put on the backburner and that we proceed to address the needs and concerns of those suffering and dying . . . In the face of the grave threat posed by HIV/AIDS, we have to rise above our differences and combine our efforts to save our people. History will judge us harshly if we fail to do so now, and right now. Let us not equivocate: a tragedy of unprecedented proportions is unfolding in Africa."

Mandela then turned to the considerable experience and knowledge that had accumulated since AIDS first emerged, which, he argued, collectively could provide powerful tools for action. "With nearly two decades of dealing with the epidemic, we now do have some experience of what works. The experience in a number of countries has taught that HIV infection can be prevented through investing in information and life skills development for young people. Promoting abstinence, safe sex and the use of condoms and ensuring the early treatment of sexually transmitted diseases are some of the steps needed and about which there can be no dispute. The experiences of Uganda, Senegal and Thailand have shown that serious investments in and mobilization around these actions make a real difference."

The speech concluded with recognition of the fact that Africa cannot fight this alone, that AIDS in Africa can only be challenged and ultimately overcome through the cooperation of people from many different levels of the global community. "The challenge," he told us, "is to move from rhetoric to action, and action at an unprecedented intensity and scale. We need, and there is increasing evidence of, African resolve to fight this war. Others will not save us if we do not primarily commit ourselves. Let us, however, not underestimate the resources required to conduct this battle. Partnership with the international community is vital. A constant theme in all our messages has been that in this inter-dependent and globalised world, we have indeed again become the keepers of our brother and sister. That cannot be more graphically the case than in the common fight against HIV/AIDS" (Mandela, 2000).

I was seated far from the stage in the huge conference hall, and though I could see the small figure of Mandela in his trademark, colorful shirt up at the front, I watched him speak via one of the large, strategically placed TV screens. His speech was frequently interrupted by applause, and after he finished, Jerry Coovadia, the South African pediatrician who had chaired the conference, told Mr. Mandela: "You cannot imagine how your speech is music to our ears. It has answered so many spoken and unspoken questions." When the conference was formally declared closed a few minutes later, there was a buzz of optimism and excitement as people filed from the hall and out into Durban's dazzling winter sunshine. "At last!" I overheard an African delegate exclaiming to her friend. "The silence has really been broken!"

The Primacy of Politics or Science?

Many people have questioned the good actually accomplished by these huge biannual International AIDS Conferences, which have been accurately described as the "trade fairs of the international AIDS industry" (Altman, 1998:239). Thousands of advocates, non-governmental organization (NGO) workers, scientists, and journalists gather in a major world city for a few fevered days of meetings and presentations. Business cards are swapped, declarations are made to loud applause, and, at the end, the exhausted delegates troop home to where nothing has changed.

But in at least one important respect, Durban was different. For all their flaws, the International AIDS Conferences are "arguably the most visible arena in which international discourses around HIV/AIDS are established and legitimized" (ibid.:241). And since Durban was the first International AIDS Conference to be held in a developing country—and the only one ever to be held in Africa, the world center of HIV, with 70 percent of all those infected worldwide—it had served as a powerful global platform for raising awareness about the sheer scale of the African epidemic as well as the totally inadequate response to it. With 24.5 million HIV-infected people, and 4 million new infections in 1999 alone, Africa's AIDS epidemic was profoundly affecting the social, economic, and demographic underpinnings of the continent's attempts to develop (UNAIDS, 2000). And by the year 2000, it really was, as Mandela had powerfully argued to his international audience, time for action.

On the basis of the new discourse promulgated at Durban, significant action did indeed follow on from the conference. A new paradigm had been established, and although Durban was not the only event contributing to what amounted to a shift in global AIDS policies, it certainly represented a watershed in the history of the African AIDS epidemic. The conference provided a huge political boost in particular to scaling up the provision of antiretroviral therapy (ART) for African people living with

AIDS. Subsequently, the establishment of the Global Fund to Fight AIDS, Tuberculosis and Malaria in January 2002, as well as enormous increases in funding from the U.S. government and the Bill and Melinda Gates Foundation, provided much of the financial basis for implementing the scale-up of these services throughout Africa.

A key observation about this process is that these changes were brought about not so much by an avalanche of scientific innovation at Durban—there had been no revolutionary discoveries announced for either the prevention or the treatment of AIDS—but rather through a simple recognition by many top level actors that it had become politically unacceptable to continue with the general abandonment of Africa to HIV. A tipping point had been reached at which, politically speaking, there was now more to lose by inaction than there was to gain. In his speech, Mandela had referred to the "dispute about the primacy of politics or science" in relation to the unresolved debate in South Africa regarding the relationship between HIV and AIDS. But this idea of the primacy of politics or science can also be applied to the transformations that followed the Durban conference in terms of developing political will and establishing global financing mechanisms to tackle AIDS. There can be little doubt that it was politics and not science that had primacy in bringing about this all-important transition.

If politics was driving the changes, what, therefore, was the role of science in addressing Africa's AIDS epidemic? I had attended the Durban conference as a delegate from Uganda, where I was working as a behavioral scientist with the British-funded Medical Research Council (MRC) Programme on AIDS. My own contribution to the meeting had been a presentation of data from a community-based HIV prevention intervention trial on which I had been working in the southwestern rural district of Masaka for the previous four years (Kinsman et al., 2000). My colleagues and I did not know at that stage whether the intervention had had any effect, so my presentation had focused on basic issues of training and support for community AIDS educators, programmatic sustainability, and condom distribution strategies. My general thrust was simply—just as Mandela had also pointed out—that these things *can* be done if there is sufficient will, money, and organization to do them.

Uganda had featured prominently throughout the conference, with many speakers praising the country's efforts. Uganda has the longest history of AIDS of any African nation, and its national AIDS Control Programme mounted a campaign very early on in the epidemic, since when HIV prevalence has fallen dramatically. While prevalence among pregnant women attending two hospitals in Kampala was estimated at 29 percent in 1992, for example, it had fallen to 10 percent and 12 percent respectively by 1999; similar prevalence patterns were also being reported from most other parts of the country (ACP, 2000:4). Furthermore, one of my MRC colleagues had presented in Durban the very first data from the entire African continent showing a significant decline in HIV incidence[1] in a general population. Like my own data, his had also been recorded in Masaka district (Mbulaiteye et al., 2000). For an AIDS scientist, these were data at their most exciting: evidence clearly indicating that things were improving. Conference delegates were watching and listening, a sign that information and ideas were being exported from Uganda to the rest of Africa. By the closing sessions, there was some pride to be had in wearing a conference name badge on which one's country was identified as "Uganda".

Politics may have had primacy at Durban, therefore, but science was certainly playing its role too. When I returned to Masaka, however, my faith in the value of science for AIDS control—or at least for HIV prevention—was shaken. Analysis of the dataset from the HIV prevention trial that I had been working on was finally completed a few months later, and it became apparent that our work had been in vain: the interventions[2] had had absolutely no impact on HIV incidence. The Masaka Intervention Trial (MIT) had been a large—and I believed well conducted—project, with a volunteer, community-based workforce of 550 people. We had recorded over 80,000 HIV prevention educational activities, 390,000 individual attendances at these activities, and the treatment of 12,000 cases of sexually transmitted diseases. Over 13,000 study participants had been interviewed, bled for serological assessment, and then followed up for an average of three and a half years for the evaluation (Kinsman et al., 2002; Kamali et al., 2003). If this degree of effort and intensity had failed to have a demonstrable impact on HIV, it was hard to imagine what could.

Two points emerged in my mind from this. First, Mandela had presented the conventional wisdom in Durban—which had accrued, in part, out of the Ugandan experience—when he said that "the experience in a number of countries has taught that HIV infection can be prevented through investing in information and life skills development for young people. Promoting abstinence, safe sex and the use of condoms and ensuring the early treatment of sexually transmitted diseases are some of the steps needed and about which there can be no dispute." In other words, he was saying, simply put, "we know what works." But the evidence we had produced in Masaka now suggested that the situation was far more complicated than this. The solid ground "about which there can be no dispute" was no longer quite as solid as it had seemed.

The second point was perhaps even more galling. As will be detailed in Chapter 6 of this book, very limited attention was paid to the findings from the Masaka study, or to their broad implications for HIV prevention in the country—either in Uganda or further afield. This was in spite of the study being a rare and rigorous evaluation of two widely adopted HIV prevention strategies. Of course, evidence of intervention success is much more exciting than evidence of failure, but it is equally important to understand the causes of failure, and then to address those causes. In this case, however, our findings were more or less completely ignored, and it was my wish to understand how and why this happened, that formed the starting point for this book.

The initial plan when I started work on the book in March 2003 was to examine the evolution of AIDS control in Uganda specifically from the perspective of research. By using an anthropological approach to investigate the means by which particular research projects had, or had not, contributed to policy changes, I hoped to be able to make some sense of what had happened to the Masaka study. I soon realized, however, that this would provide only a partial picture. More would be gained if I used a similar anthropological strategy also to examine the evolution of particular policies, to see what, in addition to research, had influenced them. Thus, I would be looking at the broad issue of AIDS control in Uganda from opposite directions: from the perspective of research (the MIT), and from the perspective of policy (through which I would focus on behavioral HIV prevention, and the scale-up of ART provision). I also planned to include an additional investigation into the process through which the need for an AIDS control policy in Uganda was recognized in the first place.

Two important points should be noted here. First, the policies to be discussed in the book are strategic, concerned with the broad approaches to HIV prevention or the provision of ART. The book is not concerned with the more technical policies to do with such issues as drug regimens or treatment algorithms. Second, it was clear from the start that both policy and research are the products of influences and processes working at many different levels. Thus, as explained in further detail below, a multilevel approach would be necessary in order to paint the fullest possible picture.

The overall objective of this book, therefore, is *to identify and explain the key influences and processes that have guided AIDS control in Uganda, from the start of the epidemic up until 2005.*[3] The specific research questions can be divided into two categories, one looking at the issue from the perspective of policy and the other from the perspective of research. Each empirical chapter addresses one or more of each of these specific questions, with the overall objective of the book running as a theme throughout.

The policy-related questions include:

1. How has AIDS control policy evolved in Uganda? Which events, at which levels, have been especially influential in this evolution, and which actors have most influenced policy formation?
2. How has international level policy impacted the development of Ugandan national policy—and vice versa?

The research-related questions include:

3. To what extent has research played a role in policy development at national and international levels? Which evidence has been used, and how?
4. What has been the rationale for conducting particular research projects on AIDS control in Uganda? What has been the reaction— from fellow scientists, policy makers, practitioners, and the target populations—to the results? What has been the impact of the findings subsequently on research, policy, and practice?

Methodological Issues

The experience of living and working in Masaka between 1996 and 2001 planted the seeds for the questions tackled in this book, and provided much of the initial raw material and understanding of the subject. Once I had started work on the project, I finalized the research questions and then began formal data collection with respect to the policies and the study concerned.

My overall methodological strategy was to follow what could be described as the life stories of three AIDS control policies and of one research project as they evolved, taking into account the respective inputs of actors from many different geographical areas and from different periods. The use of life stories in anthropology usually applies to individuals, with a narrator giving an account of his or her life, and thereby telling "what you must know about me to know me" (Linde, 1993:20). The approach here adapts the principle by taking a policy or a research project to be an individual, if very complex, entity that can only be really known through the eyes of the various actors who have shaped it, and through their understanding of how it has become what it is over the course of time. Thus it is historicized: presented and interpreted as a product of particular historical developments.

Part of the methodological inspiration for my approach has come from the Overseas Development Institute (ODI), Britain's leading independent think tank on international development and humanitarian issues. For a number of years now, researchers from the ODI have recognized that underutilization of evidence frequently hampers development policy and practice. As part of the process of bridging this gap, the ODI recommends that research into the research-policy relationship looks both from the perspective of policy (to assess the role of research in clear policy shifts) and from the perspective of research (to assess the policy impact of specific research projects) (ODI, 2004a:6). This book follows that approach; and as such, it could be described as a historical, multilevel reconstruction of AIDS control in Uganda. Below, I examine some of the methodological issues that I encountered during the process of data collection, analysis, and writing.

The study includes analysis of two main types of data. These are (i) documentary material from libraries, archives (institutional as well as personal), and the Internet and (ii) material collected during interviews conducted explicitly for this study, between 2003 and 2005, which I have been able to verify and substantiate during subsequent working trips to Uganda. Most of my research has therefore been based on what other people have written or told me, and I have sought to reconstruct events through this. Consequently, the empirical chapters that follow should not be seen as "an objective representation aimed at complete empirical coverage" (Beuving, 2006:56), or, as the founder of modern history, Leopold von Ranke, famously put it, "how it really was" (Ranke, 1824; cited in Arnold, 2000:36). Rather they are presented as the closest fit to actual events that I have been able to produce.

Returning to the two types of data that I have used: the advantage of the first—documents—is that they were produced "at the time," which means that the contents do not suffer from the treacherous historiographical practice of presentism. In other words, they have not been reanalyzed with the benefit of hindsight, with present-day ideas or perspectives anachronistically introduced into them.[4] I have files full of faded, yellowing papers collected during the late 1980s and throughout the 1990s, representing a veritable gold mine of historical information about AIDS in Africa. Yet it has struck me how easy it is to skim-read this material, since so much of what was written then seems to be so obvious now. Could people seriously have questioned whether HIV is transmissible from women to men? Is it not obvious that belief in the potential efficacy of condoms would increase the chance of people using them? But that is a presentist mental approach that does not give this material the credit it deserves. After all, at the time, these were cutting-edge research issues. The knowledge that AIDS professionals collectively currently possess has grown so fast that what was considered a few years ago to be radical and new is now taken completely for granted. If viewed carefully, these older documents can therefore open a window directly onto a former world, providing a bird's eye view of an earlier era in the particular life story being discussed.

Having said that, careful viewing and analysis is essential, as it cannot be assumed that the authors of these documents were necessarily neutral as they wrote. The information included cannot therefore be taken as simple, straightforward fact. As Furay and Salevouris (1988:223) argue, a critical approach is required when reviewing any such historical material, since one is "not study[ing] the events of the past directly, but the . . . interpretations of those events." Arnold (2000:78) takes the point further, suggesting that "sources are not innocent; their voices talk to certain ends, intend certain consequences. They are not mirrors of past reality, but events in themselves."

In a similar vein, the second type of data used in this book—interview material—must also be viewed critically. Bourdieu (1977) outlined his epistemological critique of the information derived during social scientific interviews in three points; these could apply whether the research relates to either a present-day or a recent historical issue. First, he suggests that much of an interview may remain at a level at which the basic assumptions that constitute the sine qua non of what is being discussed remain unstated. The very essence of the issue at hand is therefore avoided, potentially leading to a shallow or simply incorrect interpretation. Second, since the discussion is usually initiated by the researcher, it will flow as an outsider-oriented discourse, which means that the respondent may presume the researcher to be relatively unfamiliar with the topic, and especially so if the questioning appears to be uninformed. Hence the discussion may remain at a general level, eschewing potentially important details. Third, informants may wish to impress the interviewer with their mastery of the issue in question, which can lead to a tendency to dwell on the extremes of the range of possibilities on the topic—the "most esteemed or reprehended" (ibid.:19). This can lead to a skewed or biased dataset.

Strong as these points are, they are not necessarily fatal to research that uses interview material. Jenkins (1992) points out that most sociologists and anthropologists tend to be wide-ranging in their techniques for data collection, adopting what he describes as a "cheerful promiscuity of method" (ibid.:55). Such triangulation reduces the reliance on potentially misleading interview material; through the extensive additional use of documentary data, as well as information garnered from different levels, I have taken such a cheerfully promiscuous approach during the research for this book. Thus one type of data either supports what emerges from another or frames it in another light. But even if social scientists do decide to rely primarily on interview material for their work, Jenkins argues that

Bourdieu "overstates the case massively," and he questions "the degree to which the testimony of research subjects is, by definition, unreliable" (ibid.:56). In other words, care must be taken with such material, but it can still be used as an effective source.

Nonetheless, the material presented over the following chapters concerns very complex phenomena—the life histories of policies for AIDS control and of a large AIDS research project—which means that conflicting views and interpretations of events will inevitably arise among those who have been involved. No single account could satisfy everyone. Furthermore, while I have sought to reduce bias in analysis and interpretation to an absolute minimum, what I have written in this book is inevitably shaped to some extent by my own prejudices and preconceptions. As such, I make no universal claims about what is presented over the following pages. Rather, it should be seen simply as my interpretation of events based on data that I believe to be valid and reliable.

In his speech, Nelson Mandela made reference to "this inter-dependent and globalised world," a recognition of the many different geographical and professional arenas that play a role in a phenomenon as complex as AIDS control in Africa. Given this, I decided right at the start of this project that the only way to study my topic effectively was to take a multilevel perspective as a conceptual and methodological framework (van der Geest et al., 1990). Thus, the data collection process would require interviews with, and observations of people from, a wide range of backgrounds, living and working in many different settings. The intention has been to give voice to the actors at three different levels—international, national, and local—through which it is hoped to develop an understanding of their various emic perspectives[5] of the particular issue under discussion. For example, although the financing and much of the ostensible power originates at the international level, it will become clear over the course of the book that the relationship between levels is often based on a surprising degree of interdependence. The international actors need the national and local level actors to sustain their legitimacy just as much as the local level actors need funding from "above." A more detailed theoretical consideration of the multilevel perspective is given in Chapter 2, which highlights the importance of these relationships and linkages. The three levels are merely introduced here.

The term "international" refers here primarily to people working at the centers of research and policy making that give much of the direction to AIDS control activities for developing countries. These centers include such places as the World Health Organization (WHO) and United Nations Joint Programme on HIV/AIDS (UNAIDS), as well as the London School of Hygiene and Tropical Medicine—the individuals employed by these institutions could be described as belonging to the global elite of AIDS professionals. I chose to include people for interview at this level who are not based in Uganda but who nonetheless have insights and knowledge into particular aspects of the Ugandan AIDS epidemic. They primarily comprised social scientists, epidemiologists, physicians, and policy makers; and I met them either by appointment at their respective offices or opportunistically at scientific conferences. This fieldwork took place between July 2003 and June 2004.

For the national and local level research, I spent an intensive period in Uganda between August and December 2004, supplementing the basic foundation I had built around my research topic developed during the five years I lived in Masaka between 1996 and 2001. At the national level (which refers essentially to Kampala, where decisions are taken for Uganda as a whole), I spoke with people in the Ministry of Health, a number of NGOs, the Makerere University Institute (now School) of Public Health, the Centers for Disease Control, private consultancy firms, and with journalists.

The local level is defined here as the three contiguous districts of Masaka, Ssembabule, and Rakai,[6] and it includes the district capitals as well as the more remote rural areas (see map on page xv). At this level, I interviewed health care providers, NGO workers, local political and religious leaders, numerous ordinary people with no direct professional relationship to the issue at hand, and fieldworkers employed by medical research organizations. My travel around the local area was greatly facilitated by my driver, Ssalongo Mugerwa, who—due to my limited understanding of the vernacular, Luganda—also acted as an invaluable linguistic and cultural interpreter.

I have subsequently made several other working visits to Uganda, all of which focused in one way or another on social aspects of ART or of HIV testing and counseling. In addition to conducting the work, these trips (between 2005 and 2009) have provided me with the opportunity to substantiate and check various issues with some of the same people whom I had previously interviewed during my earlier fieldwork.

Altogether I formally interviewed 114 people for this study, some of them more than once. All could be described as knowledge-rich within at least one of the areas I was investigating. Of my respondents, 30 worked at the international level and 31 at the national level, while 53 were Masaka-based. It is important to note, however, that some people straddle different levels and I have categorized each individual here into just one. I also made extensive notes from innumerable informal meetings and conversations held at each of the three levels. Depending on the setting, respondents were selected on a convenience basis—either I already knew them or was given an introduction—with subsequent snowball sampling where appropriate. One of the reasons for there being more interviews in Masaka than at the national or international levels, for example, was the relative ease of snowballing within that smaller community.

My overall objective during interviews—which ranged in length from 20 minutes to a full evening—was to collect a maximum variation of perspectives (Hardon et al., 1994:266) on the evolution and mechanics of AIDS control in Uganda. Interviews were mostly conducted face-to-face, but some had to be done over the telephone for logistical reasons; and I always had a set of specific questions written out for each respondent. I did, however, allow myself to use and adapt these questions quite freely according to the turn a particular interview was taking, making these, in the truest sense, semistructured interviews. Most of my respondents, from all three levels, were apparently candid and uninhibited; and although I did encounter some challenging respondents, there was not a single case of outright refusal to take part.

Depending on the type of respondent and the context, I would either request that the interview be recorded (some international level respondents explicitly did not want to be recorded) or I would take notes and write these up within hours, maintaining as far as possible the respondent's precise turn of phrase. Minor editing has been necessary in places in order to make the text more readable—for example, removing unnecessary repetition, as well as "ums" and "ers"—although I have sought at all times to remain faithful to what I understood to be the original meaning.

The issue of protecting respondents' anonymity—or not—has proven to be somewhat complex in the writing of this book. From a multilevel perspective, it is striking how the desire for anonymity increases with the respondent's level. I faced several interview situations with senior government or UN officials who said they would have to receive special authorization or were otherwise very reluctant to go on the record with me. At the lower, more local levels, however, the need for anonymity becomes less relevant. Indeed, van der Geest (2003) describes how several of the old people he interviewed for a study on old age in rural Ghana were actively disappointed when their names did not appear in the book that he wrote about them. It is possible, therefore, that some of my own respondents might also regret that their names are not given next to the words that they spoke. However, given the sensitive political nature of some of the interviews, as well as the positions of some of my respondents, it seemed fair to stick to a standard and simple rule of thumb that applies across the board: if I have been unable to verify with someone that what I have written accurately represents what they told me, I have not named them. Further, I have not named anyone whose permission I did not have to do so.

This rule does not apply to people named and quoted in other documentation, or to people who are quoted as speaking in a public forum, since whatever they said is already in the public domain. Furthermore, I have given relevant professional details of a number of respondents, though not enough to make identification possible.

A final note is due here concerning my writing style for this book. Given that a number of different disciplines and areas of expertise are involved—from the recent history of Uganda to the epidemiology of AIDS to the politics of international health and research—it is likely that some readers may be familiar with certain of these areas but not with others. In order to make the material accessible to as wide an audience as possible, I have therefore held in mind during the writing process a person whom I would identify as an "intelligent ignoramus." My model reader knows little of a given subject, but is bright enough nonetheless to pick up the thread quickly to the point where she can offer valuable insights and critiques into the work. I saw my own task during the writing as providing as clear a presentation of the material and its analysis as possible, both by avoiding "unintelligible 'thick description' and esoteric jargon" (van der Geest and Hardon, 2006) and by providing notes to explain any technical terms that may not be widely understood. Through this I have sought to make the reader's task as straightforward as possible.

The Anthropologist as Both Actor and Observer: Conflicting Roles?

My own relationship with Uganda had broadly positive methodological implications for fieldwork in the country. In other words, the fact that I had once been an AIDS research actor in the country facilitated my subsequently becoming an AIDS control observer. I still had a reasonable social and professional network from my "acting" days when I returned for fieldwork in 2004, and I was also fortunate to have a couple of well-placed contacts in Kampala who provided me with the details of potential interviewees, as well as permission to use their names as references. This helped enormously to facilitate meetings, since people in key ministry, research, and NGO positions are constantly beset by academics, NGO officials, and journalists from abroad who want to come and interview them about various aspects of the Ugandan AIDS success story. Many are consequently wary of yet another intrusion into their working space, and the introductions I received as well as my former work with a reputable research organization greatly assisted in the opening of doors.

With respect to the writing itself, however, my own presence in the text is perhaps somewhat more complicated. On the one hand, it seems unreasonable to maintain that the anthropologist's appearance in his own writing is inherently problematic. I do not hold to the view that one's presence necessarily "[gets] in the way of what we should be reporting about [by] introducing noise," even if it can, "at worst, [engage us] in the self-indulgent practice called 'vanity ethnography'" (Law, 2000:7). Rather, I would argue that qualitative data cannot be disconnected from the person who has collected it, since the researcher's background, character, and status inevitably shape the process by which the material is gathered, internalized, and then interpreted (Clifford and Marcus, 1986). Just as epidemiological research papers usually provide precise details of the particular statistical packages employed for analysis, failure by the anthropologist to present any equivalent details of himself could reasonably result in the charge of claiming "the god-trick of seeing everything from nowhere" (Haraway, 1991:189). Any such pretense of omniscience would be highly misleading.

That said, my presence in parts of the book—specifically Chapter 6, which focuses on a research project in Masaka to which I devoted five years of my life—is somewhat precarious, since I am not simply an observer and interpreter of events. Rather, I appear in this chapter both in my former role as an actor *and* in my subsequent role as an observer and interpreter of the events that I once acted in. While I am not the first AIDS social scientist to work in such a way (see, for example, Farmer [2001] and Campbell [2003]), this nonetheless presents a potential methodological pitfall, since my own participation in the events in question could well impede my interpretation of what happened—especially since I was so personally disappointed with the outcome of our work. In an attempt to reduce the risk of seriously biased interpretation, I have had to make a conscious effort to stand back while writing, just as the French mathematician and religious philosopher Pascal said he did: "I cannot judge of my work while doing it. I must do as the artist, stand at a distance; but not too far" (cited in Bourdieu, 1999:8). Bourdieu's thoughts on the objectification of the act of objectification (Bourdieu, 1992:30–41)—that is, seeking first to analytically observe the processes relevant to the research topic, and then also seeking to scrutinize the analytical stance itself—have been useful in this regard. As with Pascal, I have been assisted by the passage of time, which has provided some of the distance necessary to enable me to judge the work I was involved with, or at least to interpret the processes that accompanied it rather more dispassionately than I could have done at the time.

One of my explicit intentions in undertaking this book was to try to transform the frustration that arose first out of the failure of the Masaka study to demonstrate any effect, and then out of the widespread apathy that met this lack of effect. Part of the means by which I attempted to turn these feelings into something more positive was to seek to develop an understanding of what was driving the decision makers to move in the ways that they did. In other words, by becoming an observer I hoped to resolve some of the complex issues that had arisen while I had been an actor. Only by doing this could I move on professionally. Therefore, as well as investigating the issues at hand, this book in a certain respect also describes my own journey.

Outline of the Book

The book includes seven chapters, with the first two offering background and theoretical context. The present chapter has given the introduction to the research topic, the research questions, discussion of methodological issues, and brief reflections on the anthropologist as both actor and observer. Chapter 2 provides details of the three major theoretical concepts and themes that will appear throughout the course of the book. These include (i) the multilevel perspective; (ii) the construction, nature, and use of evidence; and (iii) the links between research, policy, and practice. Collectively, this will help place the empirical chapters of the book into a wider context.

As explained above, I examine the research-policy relationship both from the perspective of policy (to assess the role of research in clear policy shifts) and from the perspective of research (to assess the policy impact of a specific research project). As such, chapters 3, 4, and 5 of this book take up the perspective of policy, by presenting the evolution of three particular AIDS control policies in Uganda. Chapter 3 discusses the early epidemic in the Masaka area and Kampala, up until 1986, when it was recognized that a national policy response to the burgeoning epidemic was actually necessary. Chapter 4 deals with the evolution of behavioral HIV prevention policy between 1986 and 2004, and Chapter 5 presents a history of treatment policy for people with AIDS in Uganda from the late 1980s up until 2005, with a particular focus on ART. The way evidence was used to support policy shifts is of primary concern here, though political and other influences are also examined.

Chapter 6, by contrast, looks at matters from the opposite perspective—that of research—by examining the life story of an HIV prevention study conducted in Masaka with which I was personally involved. The study is placed into its broad scientific and political context, its results are explained, and reaction to the findings from people in various different settings is then examined.

Chapter 7 concludes the book, with an analysis of the various threads presented in the empirical chapters. Taking the multilevel perspective as a basis for discussion, I focus first on the complex relationship that has been observed between AIDS research and AIDS policy making in Uganda. I then conclude with an analysis of the major factors that have guided AIDS control policy and practice in the country over the course of the epidemic.

2

Key Themes and Concepts

Introduction

Three interlinked theoretical themes and concepts run throughout this book in its endeavor to understand the key influences and processes that have guided AIDS control in Uganda over the course of the epidemic. These are (i) the multilevel perspective; (ii) the construction, nature, and use of evidence; and (iii) the links between research, policy, and practice.

By presenting the relevant literature and debates, this chapter provides a conceptual foundation for the empirical material that follows. It will be helpful to bear in mind throughout the chapter that although the three topics can be taken as independent entities, they can also be seen as very closely related. Indeed, their power, both methodologically and analytically, is substantially increased when considered as interrelated phenomena—as they are throughout this book—rather than as three separate ones. For example, it is only really possible to understand the evolution of a national AIDS control policy within the context of a multilevel framework that also takes into account international and local influences. Equally, one needs a thorough conceptual understanding of evidence in its various guises in order to appreciate any attempt to produce Evidence-Based Policies (EBPs).

Another point to remember is that each of the three topics are phenomena that have evolved over time—none have remained as static entities since they first emerged in the literature, and doubtless they will continue to evolve conceptually in the future. They must therefore be seen as work in progress, and whatever understanding we may have of them today cannot be considered as final. As with the empirical material presented in the following chapters, the use of a historical approach may be the most effective means of placing the subject of investigation into its full context.

(i) The Multilevel Perspective

A multilevel perspective has been adopted by researchers from a number of different social science disciplines—both quantitative and qualitative—with the intention of guiding their work conceptually, methodologically, and/or analytically. Researchers who take on this approach do so for its capacity, one way or another, to act as a heuristic tool that can help identify determining factors and explanations for what is taking place within the parameters of a given study topic. But with researchers from many different disciplines using the multilevel perspective, there is also great diversity in its definition.

On the quantitative side, a multilevel perspective has been used to assist in a wide range of epidemiological, geographical, sociological, and public health research projects. It is usually taken within the context of a statistical analysis, and the levels may include, for example, individual and ecological (Jones et al., 1991); personal and community (Matteson, et al., 1998); "society, groups, individuals, organ systems, cells, and genes" (Diez-Roux, 2000:187); and "data that are nested within individuals, such as repeated measures and multiple responses" (Demers et al., 2002:417). Such a variety of different types of levels shows how malleable the concept can be to circumstance—with all the advantages and disadvantages implicit within that fact.

Relatively few qualitative social scientists have explicitly adopted a multilevel perspective in their work,[1] but they too have tended to take the principle to suit the particular needs of their work. The rise of critical medical anthropology[2] during the mid-1980s was in part facilitated by an early use of the multilevel perspective, with Baer et al. (1986) arguing that "any discussion of power relations in the delivery of health services needs to distinguish several levels in the systems of advanced capitalist and Third World nations" (ibid.:96). They suggested that these levels—each of which incorporated its own discourse, its own emic view of the world—would include the following:

1. The macro-social, defined primarily by the capitalist world system;
2. The intermediate-social, which could include a given health institution's policies;
3. The micro-social, such as the physician-patient interaction; and
4. The individual, incorporating, for example, the patient's experiential response to illness.

With just a single factor at the highest level—world capitalism—determining everything beneath it, this is a two-dimensional, purely *vertical* multilevel perspective. Press (1990) felt it to be an unduly narrow framework, and he argued that "a heuristic model that gives excessive weight to a single element (capitalism) of a single (macro) level of explanation may not be as useful as one that utilizes a multi-level, multi-element approach" (ibid.:1001). His intention was to avoid "a monofocal approach to causal explanations" (ibid.:1002), which meant that other potentially important variables should also be included. Thus, "each level [would] consist of multiple causal sub-elements" (ibid.:1003). These could theoretically include any number of possible factors in any number of different definitions of "level," but he suggested nationalism, Islam, and Christianity at the highest level; community type, local economy, and ethnic identity at the local level; and roles, social support, as well as the world views of participants in a clinical interaction at the individual level. By taking into account the many and varied phenomena that exist globally, locally, and individually, he effectively expanded each of the levels *horizontally*.

Van der Geest et al. (1990) agreed with this line of thinking, pointing out that in an increasingly interdependent world, an anthropologist will gain only limited insights if she confines her work to the village community—the discipline's traditional domain. They insisted that "the object of research should not be isolated but rather seen as linked to 'higher' and 'lower' levels of social organization. [This] could, therefore, also be called a 'linkages perspective'" (ibid.:1026). Such linkages can be both vertical and horizontal, the latter incorporating a multisectoral perspective of each level.

Four important points emerge from this linkages perspective. First, there is no such thing as a one-way flow of ideas and communication. Rather, a thought or an impulse can move from the lower to the higher levels just as they can from the higher to the lower; and if conditions are right, the flow can also become circular (ibid.:1026). In such a case, events at the lower, local level may influence events at the national level, which subsequently can then affect the local situation again. Such a process can be facilitated when key individuals move between and understand the discourses of two or more levels. This could include, for example, a Minister of Health who is in regular contact with colleagues at the World Health Organization; or the Medical Superintendent of a district hospital who has been friends with the Minister since long before they became professionally connected. Both formal and informal links between the levels can therefore influence key events and decisions.

Second, there is invariably a degree of internal diversity within categories. Sciortino's study of health personnel in Java (Sciortino, 1992) illustrates the heterogeneity that can exist within a group that may appear at first sight to be clearly defined and discrete. She shows how the people who constitute a category—for example, patients attending a clinic, or nurses at that same clinic—do not necessarily or inevitably share the same concerns, or have the same stake in a given issue. This means that the links both between and within levels are likely to be complex and, quite possibly, difficult for a researcher to fully analyze and understand.

Third, linkages are not restricted only to the spatial realm—the vertical and the horizontal. Linkages also take place chronologically, so it may be useful to consider "phenomena . . . in their development through time" (Van der Geest et al., 1990:1026). This temporal linkage approach was adopted by Sciortino, who pointed out that "too often social phenomena have been presented as being in an eternal present, preventing a deeper understanding of the changes that have occurred" (Sciortino, 1992:7). Her study therefore sought, in part, to determine how the role of contemporary nurses in Java was a product of—or how their role was *linked* to—preceding historical developments.

The fourth point concerns not so much linkages themselves, but rather the missing links between levels. Horizontally, these could involve the relationship between traditional and biomedical health workers, or between the public and the private health care sectors, while vertically, missing links may well be found between national policy makers and local-level implementers. Temporally, it may be possible to identify missing links in a health policy, if, for example, a new national government seeks to draw a line under the political agenda of its predecessor.

These points all indicate the potentially substantial benefits that the multi-level perspective offers for the planning, conducting, and analyzing of anthropological work, but the approach does have its challenges. Perhaps the most difficult of these is practicality. As Sciortino explains (ibid.:9), multilevel work requires more logistical organization than single-level research—in terms of travel, organization, and preparation—and it may be more expensive, a fact that could explain why the approach is rarely used by anthropologists. One way of getting around this problem is to use different methodological approaches for different levels. In her multilevel study of nurses in Java, for example, Sciortino used secondary sources for the international- and national-level work, with a focus on historical, government, and administrative data.

A second challenge relates to the very strength of Press's and Van der Geest's multi-dimensional models: the fact that they provide for the identification and elucidation of numerous, complex links between different factors at different levels. The problem is that such complexity can simultaneously bring about "difficulty in assigning primacy to any single factor" (Press, 1990:1003): the more comprehensive the model, the harder it is to apply. Consequently, a social scientist may end up conducting an elaborate, multilevel research project, and yet be unable at the end of it to develop a clear conclusion. Duncan et al. (1998) warned about this, pointing out that complex, multilevel models "open up the possibility of interpretive confusion and overstatement of what may be validly concluded from a given body of evidence. Multilevel models undoubtedly have great potential, but . . . they need to be used carefully and cautiously" (ibid.:114).

In spite of these challenges, the multilevel perspective has still been used effectively by a number of medical anthropologists. Van der Geest et al. (1990), for example, took it as a basis for examining the concept of Primary Health Care (PHC). They showed that while there may have been "unanimous approval of PHC" when the idea was formally introduced at Alma Ata in 1978, subsequent "reports and publications on PHC programmes in many countries have made it clear that PHC can mean all sorts of things to different people in different positions in the political hierarchy" (ibid.:1025). In other words, while PHC is sometimes presented as an unambiguous concept, its meaning and purpose have in fact been contested by many of those involved in program funding, design, and implementation. This nuanced, multilevel interpretation of PHC as an idea was summed up as follows: "There is no such thing as a world-wide PHC concept. We will have to be satisfied with a non-definition. PHC is what people say it is" (ibid.:1033).

Huyts (1979; referred to in Van der Geest, 1990) also used the multilevel perspective to investigate PHC, but this time to drive his analysis of people's personal (as opposed to professional) motivations to participate in PHC programs. He showed how program participants at all different levels—whether technical advisers in international organizations, host governments, or the target population itself—react in "exactly the same way to PHC" (Van der Geest, 1990:1030). Ultimately, they all hope to gain something personally by participating. This could be a comfortable living and an interesting job for the technical advisers; reliable funding, and therefore a more dependable salary for bureaucrats and other employees of the host government; or personal benefits, such as free medicine, gifts, work, and connections for the targeted villagers. Huyts' use of the multilevel perspective highlighted how, in this one key respect, people are fundamentally similar, regardless of their professional background or level in the hierarchy. While it may perhaps sound rather mercenary, people will generally be far more inclined to participate in something, even if it is purportedly for the greater good, if they expect to benefit from it themselves.

Silva (1997) adopted a multilevel perspective in his historical study of conflicting interests and discourses about malaria control in colonial Sri Lanka, and he convincingly showed how actors at different levels held entirely different explanatory models for the same thing—malaria. The "colonial-scientific discourse," for example, focused on the ecological and immunological causes of the disease; the "leftist discourse" was concerned about the socioeconomic causes of malaria, for which it held the colonial government entirely responsible; while the "nationalist discourse" viewed malaria as "an externally introduced menace" (ibid.:207). The "peasant discourse"—promulgated by the very people most affected by the problem—was entirely removed from any sort of biomedical explanation. Indeed, the peasants had never even entertained the possibility that the fevers they experienced bore any relationship to the bite of a mosquito. One village leader went so far as to claim that malaria only became a problem in his area when the authorities started spraying with DDT. Through this analysis, we can see how "the meanings of concepts and objects, of words and institutions change as they move from one level to another" (Van der Geest et al., 1990:1026). Thus, something that may appear to be self-evident to people at one level may be entirely irrelevant or incorrect to those at another. This point has great relevance for health care innovations, such as the provision of antiretroviral therapy (ART) for AIDS patients in Africa. Over the past few years, international and national policy makers have faced pressure to initiate treatment for as many people as possible, with numbers treated as the target of paramount importance. However, numbers treated is of little relevance to the recipients of that treatment, whose primary concerns include ensuring that their drug supplies are maintained, that the drug side effects are kept under control, and that they have sufficient food to cope with the increased hunger that often accompanies ART (Hardon et al., 2007; see also van der Geest et al., 2010).

While these researchers have made explicit reference to their use of the multilevel perspective, there are also those who use it implicitly. Without actually using the terms "multilevel" or "linkages," two studies from Uganda demonstrate the importance and nature of vertical linkages in the country both for AIDS control and, more generally, for health policy. Parkhurst (2005) focuses on AIDS, and describes how Uganda's national AIDS policy has, over the course of the epidemic, been "carefully constructed" to fit in with the demands and expectations of international donors and non-governmental organizations (NGOs). It has, for example, been framed within the context of internationally fashionable programs such as poverty alleviation. Consequently the country has developed considerable "legitimacy" in the eyes of the international donor community in a way that few other African countries have managed (ibid.:573). Circular linkages are also highlighted in this case, with international agencies learning from Uganda's historical success in controlling HIV, and seeking then to apply the Ugandan model in other African nations.

Jeppsson et al. (2005) expand the view by looking both "up" and "down." Their paper examines how the Ugandan Ministry of Health is caught in something of a dilemma in its interactions with its two major partners: the global biomedical expert community on the one hand and the local community on the other. They describe how the particular type of personnel working at the Ministry[3] encourages ever-stronger links with the technical global institutions with which relations have long been so good. However, this coincides with a simultaneous "disembedding" from the local community, whose interests they are trying to serve (ibid.:317–318). With the concept of vertical linkages in mind, one can clearly see the dilemma faced by the Ministry: any attempt to re-embed themselves into the local community may also delink them to some extent from the international experts whose support has helped to bring about the very legitimacy of which Parkhurst wrote.

To summarize, one of the topics that has previously proven particularly amenable to study with a multilevel perspective has been the PHC movement: a global project targeting the poor and involving a multiplicity of actors. PHC lost much of its momentum during the 1980s and 1990s, since when AIDS has taken hold in many of those very same countries that were once the focus of PHC programs. And just as PHC was a good topic for study using the multilevel perspective, so too is AIDS control in Africa. Like PHC, AIDS has stimulated the development of a major global industry that seeks to assist poor people in poor countries, and whose governments are in turn highly dependent on foreign financial and technical aid.

As will become apparent over the course of the book, the agendas and understandings of actors involved in AIDS control at the various levels also vary enormously—just as they did with PHC. Thus, while recognizing the various difficulties inherent with it, a multilevel perspective—incorporating vertical, horizontal, and time-bound linkages—provides a useful foundation for a study of HIV control in an African country that has been the focus of considerable international interest for its efforts to control the virus.

The *vertical* links that will feature throughout the book connect the international, national, and local levels, and will follow the definitions given in Chapter 1. The *horizontal* linkages relate to the interactions of the different actors and institutions within each level; and the *time-bound* linkages take place over the course of the Ugandan AIDS epidemic, with each empirical chapter presenting a historical overview of its particular topic.

(ii) The Construction, Nature, and Use of Evidence

In the early 1990s, a paradigm shift occurred in clinical practice, with the emergence of "an outstanding advance in health care" (Fuchs et al., 2000:335). A team from McMaster University in Canada was concerned about the then current process of clinical decision making, which was based primarily on "unsystematic observations" and mere "clinical experience" (Evidence-Based Medicine Working Group, 1992:2421). The new paradigm for which they were advocating—which they named "evidence-based medicine" (EBM)—was based on the importance of "systematic observation" and "understanding certain rules of evidence" in order to facilitate a thorough interpretation of the medical literature (ibid.:2421). Treatment regimens based on EBM would be more effective, the Working Group argued, and patients would benefit greatly.

A hypothetical clinical scenario—regarding a man who has experienced a grand mal seizure and who visits his doctor for advice—was presented by the authors in order to contrast the limitations of "the way of the past" with the benefits of "the way of the future." The uncertainties of the old way would leave the man with "vague trepidation" about his risk of subsequent seizure, while his doctor's reference to appropriate literature via the new way would provide him with "a clear idea of his likely prognosis" (ibid.:2420). The appropriate use of quantitative data derived from rigorously conducted studies would, it was argued, reassure the patient and guide the clinician through diagnosis and treatment.

EBM rapidly strengthened its position in the world of clinical practice, but the concept also spread to other health-related disciplines. In 1998, the World Health Assembly endorsed the first-ever WHO resolution concerned specifically with health promotion, urging for the development of evidence-based health promotion policy and practice within the organization (WHO, 1998). Subsequently—as explained in the next section of this chapter—the importance of evidence for health policy, public health, and service delivery was also stressed in the Mexico Statement on Health Research (2004). The use of evidence therefore lies at the core of all fields of current health policy and practice, and it will be helpful here to define and conceptualize it in order to provide context for the empirical chapters that follow.

First of all, what is actually meant by the term "evidence"? One of the more straightforward and neutral definitions has been given as "the interpretation of empirical data derived from formal research or systematic investigations, using any type of science or social science methods" (Rychetnik et al., 2002:119). But there are also critical views of the concept. McQueen (2002), for example, argues that the very notion of evidence is "rightly viewed as [a] Western derived, European-American, and in many ways Western concept. [It] developed largely out of Western philosophical writings of the past two centuries and the epistemological underpinnings fostered by the development of logical positivism. The idea of evidence emerging from experimental design is a historical product of this development, with the randomised controlled clinical trial and the quasi-experimental approach largely creations of a Western literature" (ibid.:83).

The randomized controlled clinical trial McQueen is referring to (sometimes referred to as the Randomized Controlled Trial, or RCT) is an epidemiological tool[4] that features in this book, so it deserves some introduction here. As an experimental study design, the RCT is intended to provide the clearest possible evidence of the effectiveness or otherwise of a health-related intervention. Conducting an RCT involves a series of steps. The first of these is to randomly allocate study participants into either an intervention group or a control group.[5] The intervention is then implemented in the intervention group only, with the control group receiving either nothing at all, a placebo, or (for ethical reasons) another intervention that is deemed to be unrelated to the particular issue under investigation. Finally, the extent of any intervention effect is determined by measuring the changes in certain core indicators over the course of the intervention, and by comparing these between the intervention and control groups. For more details, see Hennekens and Buring (1987:178–212).

The RCT may be seen as a deductive approach to gathering evidence. Investigators start with a given hypothesis (for example, "beta-blockers can reduce the risk of heart attack"), and then they test the hypothesis experimentally to determine whether or not it is correct.[6] With their underlying principle of experimentation (as opposed to observation), RCTs stand at the summit of the hierarchy of what is widely deemed to constitute strong evidence. The authoritative Cochrane Database of Systematic Reviews—which to a large extent defines best practice concerning medical, surgical, and health promotion interventions—is based "on the best available information," which in the majority of cases is derived from RCTs (Cochrane, 2006).

There are those, however, who would challenge the assumption that the RCT is the natural culmination of attempts to produce the best evidence for medical science, or that it is "a matter of timeless logic" (Dehue, 2004:247). A brief history of the RCT shows that there were particular historical and nonscientific reasons for randomization emerging onto the medical scientific stage and subsequently becoming a central component of this powerful epidemiological technique.[7]

The first RCT was a British study of streptomycin for the treatment of pulmonary tuberculosis (TB), published shortly after World War II (Marshall et al., 1948). A previous study on guinea pigs with TB had demonstrated the dramatic beneficial effects of streptomycin, so it was felt that there was also a reasonable chance that the drug would work well for human TB patients. But in post–World War II Britain, with widespread rationing and only limited drug supplies, it was always necessary to do more with less. The British government had managed to purchase 50 kilograms of the new antibiotic from its American manufacturers—even though the efficacy of the drug was at that stage uncertain—most of which was to be used for treating British pulmonary TB patients, in the mere belief that it was effective. The rest of the shipment would be used for the world's first RCT in order to evaluate its efficacy. The investigators felt no ethical constraint in including an untreated control group within the study, since there was not enough streptomycin for every TB patient in Britain anyway. And by randomizing patients into either the control or the intervention group, investigators were "relieved" of any direct responsibility for allocating a scarce resource (Randal, 1999:11). Randomization was therefore a good solution for a difficult, very human problem.

Since the trial ended with a clear, positive outcome, with important implications for controlling a serious condition, the techniques and principles standing behind this first RCT were given wide publicity. Other medical scientists liked the approach, and the RCT was soon elevated to the top of the hierarchy of evidence, where it has remained ever since (ibid.:11). The RCT's fiftieth anniversary was celebrated in 1998, with the publication of a number of papers honoring the scientists who pioneered the development of this method of investigation (Fuchs et al., 2000; Randal, 1999).

The idea of the RCT as the most objective tool for deriving evidence about the effectiveness of a health intervention was therefore first accepted within the very particular cultural and historical context of Britain in the 1940s. But as Bijker and Law (1992:3) point out in relation to other innovative technologies and techniques, "it might have been otherwise." Just as with the wide acceptance of the QWERTY keyboard, or the development of the Internet, there was no predetermined certainty that medical research was going to lead to the invention and adoption of the RCT. The whole process was in fact contingent on historical circumstance. Once it had been taken up, however, it took on its own momentum and became widely accepted as the best and most objective means of collecting evidence of effectiveness, as per the principle of path dependency. This is defined in terms of "self-reinforcing sequences characterized by the formation and long-term reproduction of a given institutional pattern" (Mahoney, 2000:508). One consequence of such self-reinforcing sequences is that when a given pattern has become established and then starts to dominate, it can be easy to forget that it was not always this way.

It is useful to remember this history when considering the RCT in its elevated position as the gold standard epidemiological tool. Initially designed to evaluate clinical interventions, it has proven to be a highly effective tool for studies of this nature. But with the principles of EBM moving increasingly into health promotion activities, the boundaries of what is deemed appropriate for evaluation by an RCT have expanded to include behavioral interventions, including those intended to control HIV. This process has been driven by concerns about the "lack of well-designed, robust studies to evaluate the effects of [sexual behavior] interventions" (Stephenson et al., 2000:S115), and arguments that "without well designed trials of sex education, uncertainty and dogma will frustrate efforts to seek a better way forward" (Stephenson, 1999:69). More specifically, there have been suggestions that "evaluation design in this [HIV prevention and sexual health] field needs to be improved," and that there should be "more use of randomized controlled trials and the raising of publication standards by journals" (Oakley et al., 1995:479). The evidence base for maximizing the effectiveness of AIDS control activities would, it is argued, be best supplemented through wider and better use of RCTs.

However, several commentators have spoken out explicitly against this trend of using the RCT as the tool of choice for producing evidence about sexual behavior interventions. One of the more outspoken of these critics has argued that "most if not all sexual health interventions are of the sort that makes them inherently unsuitable for experimental evaluation, particularly the kind of evaluation set out by the Cochrane Collaboration" (Kippax, 2002). One of the arguments is that possible intervention target points for HIV control are not linked in "simple, demonstrable chains of causation where single factors are manipulated to produce single, easily measured outcomes" (McQueen, 2000:96). Thus it can be very hard to determine precisely which outcome measures would be relevant when evaluating the intervention in question, and also what would constitute an appropriate length of follow-up (Nutbeam, 1999). Any evidence emerging from such a study may therefore be seen as "too restrictive" (ibid.:100) and "reductionist" (Bonell, 2002:386), and may not be especially useful for policy development.

The debate about the various benefits of and problems with the RCT has sometimes been bitter, with one epidemiologist describing Kippax's antitrial critique as "recklessly arrogant" (cited in Low, 2004:435). But there are several alternative sources of epidemiological evidence, and since these are not held up as the gold standard approach, they tend to provoke less controversy. Hennekens and Buring (1987:3) subdivide epidemiology into two categories—descriptive and analytical—the first being concerned with the distribution of disease, and the second with the determinants of disease. As an experimental technique intended to determine whether a particular intervention prevents a particular disease, the RCT is clearly an analytical epidemiological approach. Likewise, the cohort study approach— in which "subjects are classified on the basis of the presence or absence of exposure to a particular factor and then followed for a specified period of time to determine the development of disease in each exposure group" (ibid.:22)—also falls into the analytical epidemiological category, although it is a passive, observational method rather than an interventionist or experimental one. It too includes an explicit comparison of exposure and disease status and can provide strong evidence of association, if not causation, between the two. By contrast, the cross-sectional survey is a purely descriptive epidemiological approach, involving just one interview with each respondent, and therefore with no possibility of follow-up that can help determine the nature of any temporal relationship between exposure and disease. Cross-sectional surveys are useful tools for producing snapshot evidence about a given disease in a given population, but they are not designed to test hypotheses and they cannot be used to demonstrate causation. Both the cohort study and the cross-sectional survey will appear later in the book as sources of evidence that have played a role in various aspects of AIDS control in Uganda.

The focus here so far has been on epidemiological evidence, but it is important to note that evidence can also take many other forms. Epidemiological studies are by their very nature quantitative exercises, following a principle outlined by the nineteenth-century physicist Lord Kelvin: "To measure is to know" (cited in Lagerros, 2009:119). But this positivist perspective was challenged by fellow physicist Albert Einstein, who suggested that "not everything that counts can be counted; not everything that can be counted counts" (cited in McKee, 2004:153). In other words, qualitative evidence can also provide insights about the inherently immeasurable, but no less important, aspects of an intervention. Among other things, these could include people's feelings and lived experiences. Price and Hawkins (2002) have developed a qualitative approach for the evaluation of sexual and reproductive health interventions, which they call peer ethnography. By using already-recognized members of the community as researchers, this amounts to a rapid appraisal approach that emphasizes the importance of having an established level of trust between researcher and respondent. The authors argue that a comprehensive understanding of factors associated with sexual and reproductive health can only be realized through research based on trust, and that such trust cannot be attained through the impersonal approach that is more or less inherent within the RCT or other purely quantitative epidemiological techniques.

A degree of tension therefore exists between those who advocate quantitative and those who advocate qualitative methods in the production of evidence. This is a tension born largely of strict but arbitrary disciplinary boundaries, whether in the field of epidemiology or in the various social sciences: people working in a given discipline rarely engage with or understand other disciplines. But there are those who point out that the wide range of existing methodological approaches should be put to full use in order to meet the demands of different situations. In other words, there is the need for a "post-positivist paradigm for health promotion research" (Tones and Green, 2004:327). As Nutbeam (1999:100) suggests, "the most compelling evidence of effectiveness comes from studies that combine different research methodologies—quantitative with qualitative. The use of a wide range of data and information sources will provide more relevant and sensitive evidence of the effects of multi-dimensional health promotion interventions than a single 'definitive' study." Tones and Green (2004:321) add that intervention evaluations should also "address process and context as well as outcomes." The argument, therefore, is not to use only quantitative methods or only qualitative methods, and to disregard other approaches. Rather, the argument is to avoid relying on just one type of evidence and instead to triangulate using a variety of complementary methodological approaches—for example, an RCT in conjunction with an ethnographic approach in the evaluation of an HIV prevention behavioral intervention.

No matter which methodological approach is used for the production of evidence, however, we shall see over the following chapters that the same evidence may be interpreted and used by different people in very different ways at different times. This is particularly notable in the policy arena, where decision makers have to juggle with many different, and sometimes conflicting, influences. Evidence is just one of these, and yet, since it carries with it the weight and authority of "objective science," it may be held up as a particularly useful means of supporting a given policy. Consequently, it can take on a remarkable elasticity of meaning as politicians seek to justify their motives for action.

(iii) Linking Evidence with Policy and Practice

Given the overall objective of this book—to identify and explain the key influences and processes that have guided AIDS control in Uganda over the course of the epidemic—an examination of the links between research, policy, and the practice of intervention implementation is of central importance. Evidence derived from research has the potential to play an important role in defining the nature of both policy and practice, but, as we shall see, the connections are by no means always straightforward.

The previous section examined the concept of evidence, so it would be helpful here to briefly discuss what is meant by the term "policy." The definitions available in the literature range from the technical to the poetic, and it would be difficult ever to produce a definition that is universally acceptable. The London-based Overseas Development Institute (ODI) defines policy as "a purposive course of action followed by an actor or set of actors" (ODI, 2004a:2)—though it could equally be argued that a purposive course of *in*action may also constitute a (probably unwritten) policy. ODI highlights the multifaceted character of policy by pointing out that it is produced not only by governments but also by international organizations, bilateral agencies, and NGOs.

Shore and Wright (1997) focus on the inherently intangible nature of policies. Adapting a metaphor from Arthur Koestler (1967), they suggest that policy is "the ghost in the machine, the force which breathes life and purpose into the machinery of government, and animates the otherwise dead hand of bureaucracy" (Shore and Wright, 1997:5). They also show how it is a somewhat elusive concept, since, as demonstrated through a multilevel perspective, a given policy can have different meanings for different categories of actors and in different places. "On close examination," they argue, "policy fragments. It becomes unclear what constitutes a policy. Is it found in the language, rhetoric and concepts of political speeches and party manifestos? Is it the written document produced by government or company officials? Is it embedded in the institutional mechanisms of decision making and service delivery? Or is it whatever people experience in their interactions with street level bureaucrats?" (Ibid.:5)

In addition to being intangible and elusive, policy is also a contested phenomenon. Yanow (1993) focuses on what a policy means, to whom, and how it attains that meaning; and she shows how a policy can mean different things to different groups of people, between whom there may be competing interests. Similarly, Walt and Gilson (1994) argue that studies of the policy process require examination of "who is likely to favor or resist [changes in] policy" (ibid.:353), since the power plays between actors can significantly determine the way and the extent to which a policy may be implemented.

Thus, the concept of "policy" embraces many different definitions and meanings. One way or another, however, they all suggest that someone—a policy maker—intends some specific sort of action or inaction as the outcome of his or her decision.

Evidence-based policy making

The means by which evidence is produced for use in such activities as clinical practice and health promotion was examined earlier in this chapter. And, as suggested, the use of evidence has by no means been restricted to these spheres, with Evidence-Based Policies (EBPs) also attaining prominence over recent years. The extent to which the principle of EBP has now been accepted is illustrated by the Mexico Statement on Health Research, which was the product of a ministerial summit on health research held in Mexico City in November 2004. Attended by health ministers and other senior representatives from 58 countries—including Uganda's then Minister of State for Health, Alex Kamugisha—the final communiqué concluded that "health policy, public health and service delivery should be based on reliable evidence derived from high quality research . . . Ignoring research evidence is harmful to individuals and populations, and wastes resources" (Mexico Statement on Health Research, 2004:1).

WHO is a central player in formulating and promoting EBPs. As a means of facilitating evidence-based policy making, the world body has established the Health Evidence Network, whose function is to provide "answers to policy questions in the form of evidence-based reports and summaries" (Health Evidence Network, 2006). National and international policy makers are also urged to follow the findings of well-respected, systematic analyses such as those found in the Cochrane Reviews (Garner et al., 2004). Furthermore, a "GRADE" approach has been developed to "grade the quality of evidence and strength of recommendations" in the development of EBPs (GRADE Working Group, 2004:1496). This assigns grades to different types of evidence, with the RCT rated "high," observational studies "low," and any other evidence "very low" (ibid.:1493). A hierarchy of evidence similar to that used in evidence-based clinical practice has therefore been produced—with experimental, quantitative studies ranked at the top—in order to inform and guide health policy decisions.

However, some observers have criticized this approach. Ankrah (1989) argued early in the epidemic that most of the AIDS research conducted in Africa had been medically oriented, even if it is in essence a social disease—and even if tackling it through effective policies will inevitably require a comprehensive understanding of its many social determinants and components. In other words, not enough of the right research had been conducted. There was, as she put it, "too much epidemiology, too little social science" (ibid.:267). Citing Kleinman (1978), she went on to suggest that dealing with the African AIDS epidemic requires taking into account not only the explanatory models of the people suffering from the disease but also the explanatory models of the professionals who are guiding the national and international response to it. If a better balance is not struck between epidemiological and social scientific African AIDS research, there is a risk that evidence-based policies and guidelines may be formulated, but these may not be well-grounded in the social realities of ordinary African people.

Furthermore, even within the disciplines of epidemiology and clinical medicine, a related critique points out that "many questions relevant to public policy makers have not yet been asked, or addressed. Moreover, a systematic review can fail to yield a research-based answer to a public policy maker's question, because high quality work has either not been done or is not locally applicable" (Lavis et al., 2004:1616). Thus it is important for a study to ask the right question in the right setting. And once that is done, it is then also important for the investigators to be able to comprehensively analyze and interpret the findings of their study in such a way that policy makers are able to act on them. However, as suggested above, unraveling causal relationships between the many dynamic variables that are involved in an intricate and multifaceted sexual health intervention is very difficult, especially within the confines of purely quantitative research methodologies. The overall result is a "lack of empirical evidence available for a government to base policies or decide on priorities, despite the large amount of research undertaken and published on the subject" (Macintyre et al., 2001:224). It is clearly ambitious to expect that truly evidence-based sexual health policies can be produced in such conditions.

A further problem is that additions to the research literature are "more usually research-producer driven rather than led by research-users' needs" (Davies and Nutley, 2002:6). Many researchers believe there is—or ought to be—a straightforward, linear relationship between research and policy, and they work under the rather optimistic conviction that their work feeds neatly into the policy process. Black (2001:275) describes this situation as one in which "a problem is defined and research provides policy options. Research is used to fill an identified gap in knowledge." However, he and several other authors have pointed out that such a model of events is not empirically grounded, with the key missing variable identified as context—whether political, financial, and/or social (Debrow et al., 2004). As Donald (2001:278) suggests, "policy decisions are almost always made in the context of money, power, and precedent." Poulos and Zwi (2005:429) take the point further, conceding that they have "come to the realization that research has, in fact, little impact on policy making."

These authors were writing about the relationship between evidence and health policy in countries such as the UK and Australia, and collectively they point to a divide between the rhetoric of evidence-based policy making and what has been observed empirically. On the one hand, there is a global trend toward accepting evidence-based policy making as the most rational and appropriate means of defining effective policies, and this is a view to which most nations currently officially subscribe. Uganda is among these, with the country's Health Sector Strategic Plan stating that "research is a critical tool for evidence-based policy and decision making. It provides an informed basis for guiding and rationalizing implementation of the health sector strategic plan" (MoH, 2000:66). The point was reemphasized in 2006, at a high-profile meeting at the Toronto International AIDS Conference, with a senior Ministry of Health official stating that "our policy in Uganda is evidence-based, [so] that if information occurs from studies, then we must incorporate the findings into our planning" (Kaiser Network, 2006:24). But on the other hand, there appears to be a host of problems inherent in putting the rhetoric of evidence-based policy making into action, with some observers arguing that the link is tenuous at best.

A great deal of AIDS research had been conducted in Uganda by the time the Mexico Statement on Health Research was produced in 2004—some of which, as we shall see, was explicitly intended to inform policy. Meanwhile, a broadly effective AIDS control policy had also been in place in the country for many years. One of the main themes of this book, therefore, will be an extension of the discussion about the link—or lack of it—between research and policy that has been held in a number of Western countries, into the context of AIDS control over the course of the Ugandan epidemic.

A model of the policy process

While current rhetoric espouses evidence-based policy making, therefore, a number of other factors also play an important role in the policy process. Given this diversity of influences, how do health policies actually emerge? Seeking to understand the policy environment is not simply an interesting intellectual exercise, but rather a prerequisite that may allow us to "operate more effectively in the promotion of policy change" (Walt, 1994:207). It therefore has potentially important practical implications.

Many authors have sought to unpack the ways and means by which policy is made, though most of the models have been developed by Western-based academics, and few are specific to health policy. The ODI has a list of 31 such theories (ODI, 2006), which incorporate a great variety of viewpoints and academic points of departure. They range from Kuhn's paradigm shift (Kuhn, 1962) to Lipsky's model of street-level bureaucrats (Lipsky, 1980), to the idea of epistemic communities (Adler and Haas, 1992).

This theoretical diversity demonstrates the very complexity of the process, but out of these 31 theories, ODI has synthesized a simple generalized model, which will be presented over the next few pages. The model (Court, 2004:16) outlines a series of stages that, one way or another, may be encountered during the policy process (see table 2.1). It is important to note that the step-by-step nature of the model does not in any way imply that events inevitably move smoothly from one to the next in a linear fashion, as clearly they do not. Equally, this is not a model that will be forced onto the empirical material presented in the following chapters. Rather, the framework is offered as a starting point for seeking to understand the complex policy processes that will emerge over the course of the book.

Table 2.1   The policy process—a simplified theoretical model

1. *Agenda Setting*: Awareness is raised of an issue or problem. If it is deemed a priority concern, it may then appear on the policy agenda;
2. *Policy Formulation*: Options for solving the problem are debated, and potential strategies are constructed;
3. *Decision making*: Decisions are made about which strategy or strategies to pursue. The policy has now been set;
4. *Policy Implementation*: The policy is implemented through activities on the ground;
5. *Policy Evaluation*: Monitoring and evaluation seeks to assess the effect and/or impact of these activities, in order to inform a future policy review. There, the policy may be amended, withdrawn, or it may remain untouched.

Source: Adapted from Court, 2004:16.

Kingdon (1984) takes the first of the model's five steps—agenda setting—and suggests that issues tend to find their way onto policy agendas when three distinct streams coincide. These include (i) the problem stream, (ii) the policy stream, and (iii) the politics stream. Many issues are likely to be circulating at any given time within the first of these—the problem stream—but an issue such as AIDS may only emerge as predominant when, for example, alarming new surveillance data on HIV prevalence is published. The second, the policy stream, includes people—such as those in an epistemic community of AIDS clinicians, scientists, or activists from NGO networks—who have putative solutions to the problem. It is important to note that different epistemic communities may have quite different views on how to solve the same problem, and at some point they are likely to be competing with each other. The third, the politics stream, is made up of government officials and politicians whose immediate concerns may not always be shared by the activists and doctors.

Within this framework, Kingdon suggests, there may be regular overlap between the problem and policy streams—in other words, activists and scientists are constantly seeking possible solutions for a given problem. Unless a window of opportunity opens, however, and the politics stream also becomes involved, an issue will probably not appear on the national or international policy agenda. At this point, in Kingdon's words, it has entered the "policy primeval soup," where it then competes with other issues for attention and funding (cited in Evans and Davies, 1999:379). In this model, research plays a contributory role, but bringing an issue onto the policy agenda is also contingent on additional, external conditions.

With an issue now on the political agenda, it is necessary to decide upon an appropriate course of action. This takes place during stages two and three of the model: policy formulation and decision making.

Evidence derived from research has a clear potential to enter into the process during these stages. A good example of how this can happen is given by Walt et al. (2003), who describe what they term as the "policy loops" that led to the widespread international acceptance of syndromic sexually transmitted disease (STD) management[8] as a means of reducing HIV incidence. As will be explained in further detail in Chapter 6, a large RCT conducted in Mwanza, Tanzania (Grosskurth et al., 1995), suggested that this strategy could reduce HIV incidence by as much as 42 percent. Walt shows how such a field-level, context-specific generation of data led "upwards" to global policy networks, where the findings were packaged so they could then be marketed and disseminated back "down" to countries all across the globe. It was by no means a straightforward process, and is characterized in the paper as "diffuse, iterative and 'looped'... [It] cannot be described as linear, rational, bottom-up or top-down, coercive or voluntary, but may display any of those characteristics at different points" (Walt et al., 2003:12, 26). What happened through this very specific, if rather convoluted process, therefore, was that syndromic STD management became established as global best practice, and policy makers throughout the developing world were then encouraged to adopt it. Thus, once it had been repackaged, the evidence from Mwanza fed directly into national-level policy formulation and decision making in countries throughout the world.

The Mwanza trial demonstrates how research can contribute to these steps in the policy process, but in some respects it is such a good example precisely because it was a highly unusual case. It is very rare that findings from a single study are so conclusive that policy makers worldwide sit up and take note. Rather, research more often has an indirect effect on the process, by introducing new directions of thought and thereby shaping the policy discourse (ODI, 2004a:2). The reason it worked so directly with Mwanza was that, as in Kingdon's model, the problem, policy, and politics streams came together in a rare convergence: the problem had been recognized, a viable solution was on offer, and the policy makers liked it. As one observer put it, "Mwanza fell into a ready made bed" (Philpott et al., 2002:199).

Viewing this from a multilevel perspective, Mwanza also provides a good example of the "exaggerated impact [that international actors can have] on research and policy processes in developing contexts" (Court, 2004:15). In the case of Mwanza—which was the product of a multinational collaborative effort, led by non-Tanzanian scientists—this multilevel aspect had a broadly positive outcome. But since much of the research conducted in Africa is conceptualized and conducted by outsiders, it may be neither "needs-oriented" nor "demand-driven" (RAWOO, 1999:13). Furthermore, donor-led research often results in a "loss of institutional memory. The turn-over of personnel in the donor community is very high, and tours of duty relatively short. This undermines continuity in the research programs and policy formulation" (van Zyl, 2003:16). In response to this critique, some of the major donors are now seeking to redress the balance through putting "greater emphasis on developing country ownership of research initiatives, and on research capacity enhancement in the south" (RAWOO, 2002:6). Through this, it is hoped that appropriate policy formulation and decision making will be facilitated.

The fourth step in the ODI model consists of implementation, the actual process of putting a policy into practice. In some respects this is the hardest step of all (Court and Maxwell, 2005:714), and it also probably has the least to do with the direct use of evidence derived from research. Implementation has been framed elegantly, if somewhat tongue-in-cheek, in terms of "a clash between the political will and the administrative won't" (O'Neil, 2005:762), though it is not always administrative intransigence that impedes policy implementation. Okuonzi points to Uganda's progressive policies for women, children, and the disabled, but suggests that "most of these policies have remained largely unimplemented because of lack of funding" (Okuonzi, 2004:1632). By contrast, Parkhurst and Lush (2004) argue that the Ugandan government has been quite shrewd with respect to implementing its AIDS control policies, by allowing nonstate actors considerable freedom to work within the broad parameters of a vaguely defined "open" policy on AIDS. The government—which has severe budget limitations—has not therefore had to bear a high proportion of the costs of implementing its own policy. In 2005, for example, just 6 percent of the annual AIDS budget of $202 million spent on AIDS in Uganda came from government coffers, with foreign donors covering the rest (UNAIDS, 2008). Through this, the government has sidestepped what would have amounted to an administrative "can't" by permitting outsiders to pay to get the job done. Research played little or no role here. Rather, this could be interpreted as straightforward, pragmatic politics.

The fifth step of the ODI's scheme, evaluation, is of course an intrinsically research-related activity, and in a perfect world, one would expect that the findings from an evaluation of a health intervention would feed back directly into a fine tuning of the relevant policy. It does not always happen in this way, however, since "political context is the most crucial issue affecting the uptake of research into policy" (Court, 2004:7).

"Political context" can be broadly defined to include issues relevant at the global scale right down to the relationships, perspectives, and incentives of the various actors in a Ministry of Health. Judith Justice (1987) took the latter level of definition in her study examining the bureaucratic context of PHC in Nepal, where she found that many PHC programs in the country had been ineffective because "they reflected the perspective and needs of the health bureaucracies involved rather than those of the local villages receiving services" (ibid.:1301). Furthermore, it was difficult for the bureaucrats to take the findings and recommendations of the PHC evaluations that had been conducted into account simply because their bureaucratic needs—the political context in which they worked on a day-to-day basis—did not permit the necessary changes to be made.

In this sense, political context at a relatively low bureaucratic level impeded an effective response to the evaluation of the PHC programs. Other studies have shown that if it is politically expedient at a higher, ministerial level—if the results of an evaluation "legitimate or sustain a predetermined position already taken by policy makers" (Moynihan, 2004:3)—the research will be included in future policy decisions. If not, it may be rejected.

Advocacy and policy

The discussion so far has been concerned largely with how research can influence policy. But it is important to note that there are also cases where research emphatically does *not* influence policy, where a particular policy is produced irrespective of whether or not supporting evidence exists. Two international-level examples of this are the United Nations' Millennium Development Goal (MDG) for AIDS, which seeks to halt and begin to reverse the spread of HIV/AIDS by the year 2015, and the WHO's '3 by 5' initiative—which sought to bring 3 million people onto ART by the end of the year 2005. The global AIDS epidemic had finally emerged onto the international political agenda by the turn of the twenty-first century, and world leaders were anxious to be seen to be doing something about it. As Putzel (2004) describes in relation to the Ugandan AIDS epidemic in the late 1980s, a threshold had been crossed and it became politically more expedient to take action rather than to continue with the status quo. WHO and other UN agencies therefore took the lead in developing these extremely ambitious targets for prevention and treatment, with a particular focus on improving conditions in heavily affected developing countries.

But those who set the MDG target for AIDS have been accused of being "profoundly naïve," and of setting an "impractical" target, with "no evidence [being used in] the setting of the strategy" (ODI, 2004b:7). The charge with respect to '3 by 5' is similar: "There was no robust evidence in the development of that target," which meant that there was consequently "great scope for wasting massive sums of money" (Court, 2004:60, 66).

There are still several years until the MDG can be fully evaluated, but the '3 by 5' strategy failed spectacularly to achieve its ambitious objective, missing the targeted 3 million patients on treatment by a full 1.7 million (UNAIDS, 2006:4). Nonetheless, though the target itself may have been missed, the strategy as a whole was a significant, if incomplete, success. Largely due to the enormous global resources that were mobilized as a result of '3 by 5,' 1.3 million people with AIDS were receiving treatment by the end of 2005—far more than before the initiative began, and far more than would have been the case in its absence. Thus, while this *non*-evidence-based policy may have failed on its own terms through not meeting its own target, it contributed enormously to the health of well over 1 million people, and thereby also provided immeasurable support to their families and communities. There may be no evidence to support a given policy, therefore, but the eventual outcome can still be very positive.

Nonetheless, it is still worth asking how, in this era of evidence-based policy making, these *non*-evidence-based policies found their ways so firmly onto the international political agenda. The MDG and '3 by 5' represent a sea change in the history of AIDS in Africa, since they constitute a successful outcome to the enormous global pressure produced by activists and advocates that grew during the late 1990s and early 2000s. Advocacy involves clearly positioning oneself and then arguing in favor of a particular cause or policy. And if done effectively—as it was in bringing AIDS into international focus during the late 1990s—it can become the linkage between social movement, knowledge generation, and political activity: "The triangle that moves the [policy] mountain" (Moynihan, 2004:18).

So how does an advocate go about embedding her empirically derived recommendations into an appropriate political and social context, and thereby moving the policy mountain? Walt et al. (2003) quote an advocate who explains succinctly how her work is done: "You don't slowly and carefully build an argument in order to convince—you start with a simple clear message to grab attention, and work down and start filling in the gaps and the explanations" (Walt et al., 2003:19). This may sound unscientific, and possibly even rather disingenuous, but there are those who argue that AIDS researchers actually bear a degree of responsibility to become advocates, and to try to ensure that their findings are put into action. As Charlie Gilks of WHO's Department of HIV/AIDS explains, "there is no other field where the opportunities to translate evidence into action are so great. Not only can researchers directly impact on policy and practice, they have a real opportunity to reduce the inequity between those who usually benefit from science and those who do not" (cited in Njoroge, 2005).

Thus there may be a degree of moral responsibility incumbent on AIDS researchers, but advocacy can become a minefield for a scientist who wishes to maintain credibility and legitimacy, as well as his reputation for being objective. Advocate-scientists run the risk of being charged with interpreting data to suit their own political perspective or value system. In the words of one observer, "[T]o the extent you are a social advocate, you're not a scientist, you lose your credibility" (Moynihan, 2004:18). An excellent example of this is given by UNAIDS, who show how "data can be interpreted in many ways, depending on how they are selected, manipulated and presented" (UNAIDS, 2004:9). According to the agenda of the individuals presenting a dataset, they demonstrate how the very same material can be used by a lobbyist for abstinence-based sex education, or an NGO seeking funding for condom promotion in secondary schools, or a program planner who simply wants to give a picture of sexual risk in the population (ibid.:9).

For a researcher who wishes to enter this treacherous world of advocacy, Moynihan suggests two principles: policy recommendations derived from research should be both *actionable* and *accessible* (Moynihan, 2004). With respect to their being actionable, one of the major challenges facing researchers who seek to influence policy is that findings are rarely clear-cut. There are usually uncertainties within the data or its interpretation, and a degree of hedging is therefore necessary in order to maintain scientific integrity. But this is unlikely to be helpful to policy makers. As UNAIDS points out, "policy makers want clear action points. Senior politicians do not want more problems, they want solutions" (UNAIDS, 2004:26). The message must therefore be distilled to its essentials in the clearest way possible in order to ensure that policy makers know what to do with it. Given the inherently political nature of policy making, findings that are presented without clear and actionable recommendations are likely to be either ignored altogether, or reinterpreted in order to legitimate a predetermined position (Moynihan, 2004:3).

With respect to accessibility, a *Lancet* editorial has argued that there is a distinct lack of "technical competence to absorb the results of research and translate them into policies" in many developing countries, and that in such contexts this is "research capacity's weakest link" (Lancet, 2001:1381). Given this fact of life, researchers need to publish their work both as technical, scientific papers in peer-reviewed journals, and also in formats that make the findings easily digestible for people without training in their given discipline (Horchler et al., 2004).

By ensuring that the recommendations that arise out of their work are both actionable and accessible to policy makers, AIDS researchers can facilitate the process of translating important evidence—produced through diverse methodological approaches, both quantitative and qualitative—into truly evidence-based policies. This does not mean that these policies will necessarily be acted upon—the administrative "won't," or a lack of funds, can always get in the way—but if researchers fail to champion their findings, they are unlikely to be taken up at all. They may then reasonably be charged with fiddling while Rome burns; and given the enormous scale of the African AIDS epidemic, this would be an untenable moral position.

3

Accepting the Unacceptable: Establishing a National Response to AIDS in Uganda

Introduction

In the early 1980s, Uganda was hit by the world's first extensive AIDS epidemic in a general population. The districts of Rakai and Masaka, just to the north of the border with Tanzania, bore the brunt of the suffering, with widespread decimation of homes and communities. But although it took several years for the country to establish a substantive policy response, Uganda was nonetheless one of the first African countries to react against AIDS—and to react with considerable success.

Things could, however, have been very different. Many of Uganda's East African neighbors mounted what could only be described as a lackluster response to AIDS during the 1980s, and there were also strong forces working within the country to inhibit any sort of policy response. There was no precedent for action, and thus the founding in 1986 of the national AIDS Control Programme (ACP) was an impressive accomplishment.

The objective of this chapter is to describe the process that culminated in the establishment of the ACP, and to identify these inhibiting forces as well as those that contributed toward the eventual policy outcome. To this end, a social history of events is presented, including material from each of the international, national, and local levels.

An important concept that will help illuminate this material is the "imagined epidemic." As the name suggests, this can be defined as the way in which the various actors involved perceive or imagine an unfolding epidemic (Streefland, 1998). The concept has previously been used in analysis of events surrounding the Black Death, as well as various plague and cholera epidemics, and its value lies in demonstrating that there are as many interpretations of events surrounding an epidemic as there are actors involved. Individuals' interpretations can be influenced by such diverse factors as rumors, memories of previous epidemics, the media, information from the medical world, and trust—or a lack of it—in the abilities of medical professionals to assist. A central tenet of the concept is that perceptions and representations play an essential role in shaping a society's response to an epidemic.

This relates to AIDS in Uganda—as elsewhere—since the epidemic was still being constructed as a social process for several years after it was first identified. Many different and competing interpretations of events were in circulation. As Sommerfeld (1994:280) notes, "epidemics need to be considered as social processes that are [both] socio-culturally and epidemiologically constructed." Such social processes may take some time, which was certainly the case in developing the broad consensus that currently prevails in Uganda, that HIV causes AIDS. In other words, literally everyone involved, at each of the three levels—international, national, and local—struggled for some time to grasp what was happening. This is an important starting point for seeking to understand the process that finally led to the establishment of the ACP.

Much of what follows is presented from the perspective of scientists who were involved in African AIDS research at the time, and especially from those based in Uganda. They provided a significant proportion of the material that fed into the social construction of AIDS in the first place; and by presenting essential information as to the extent and nature of the burgeoning epidemic, these scientists also contributed significantly to the establishment of Uganda's ACP. Indeed, Putzel (2004:22) has gone so far as to describe the "crusading role" of this small group of individuals in the country, which included physicians, virologists, and surgeons, both Ugandan and expatriate. Without their collective efforts, and without the ear of a President who was willing to listen to them, much more time would have passed before AIDS control activities commenced in Uganda.

Uganda's War against All Diseases—and against Tanzania

The late 1970s was a period of great hope in the world of international public health. The Alma Ata Declaration was signed in 1978, promising "Health for All" by the year 2000, through the establishment of the Primary Health Care (PHC) movement (WHO, 1978); and there was increasing evidence that smallpox had finally been vanquished. No new case of the horrific disease had been identified anywhere in the world since late 1977, and eradication now seemed virtually assured (WHO, 1977).

This global feeling of optimism was reflected by Ugandan President Idi Amin when he introduced his 1977 Venereal Disease Decree:

"This is a military government, and a government of action . . . The Life President wants to lead not only rich people but people who are literate, intelligent, peaceful, happy, healthy, and strong . . . He has fought the Economic War[1] and won it. He has now set out to fight a war against all diseases (cited in Lyons, 1999:109).

But a series of entirely unrelated political events were unfolding, that would extinguish any hope that Uganda's war against all diseases would be won—and that would also provide a huge challenge to the aspirations of the Alma Ata Declaration itself. President Amin kept control of the country during his eight-year presidency through a ruthless divide-and-rule strategy that pitted northerners against southerners, and by using clan loyalties to keep different groupings within the army vying for his favors. However, a string of state-sanctioned assassinations in 1977 had left certain of his military allies deeply angry, and Amin decided that the best way to shore up flagging support from within the army was to engage his troops in a foreign adventure (Fountain, 1992:53). The border with Tanzania had long been a point of contention between the two countries: the straight, East-West line that separates them was drawn at the Congress of Berlin in 1885, and it denies Uganda the 1,800 square kilometer Kagera Salient that it could otherwise quite easily consider to be its own (see map on page xv). Amin decided that annexing Kagera would provide the necessary stimulus to reunite his military support base.

In October 1978, Uganda therefore sent 3,000 troops across the Tanzanian border. These soldiers included Amin's much-feared Suicide Battalion—who were based at the barracks in Masaka, 80 kilometers north of the border—and his Simba Battalion from Mbarara, 100 kilometers to the west; and they left behind them "a trail of rapes, murders and looting" as they went about the occupation and annexation of Kagera (ibid.:53). The Tanzanian authorities did not sit idly by, and within days, President Julius Nyerere had assembled a substantial force to respond. Geography dictated that the Tanzanian return invasion of Uganda would inevitably pass through the districts of Rakai and its neighbor to the north, Masaka, and this productive agricultural area bore the rage of thousands of Tanzanian troops and Ugandan rebels in early 1979, as they fought their way toward the capital city Kampala and, subsequently, the ousting of Idi Amin. Shortly before he fell, Amin complained that the invasion forces—which included the 207th battalion of the Tanzanian People's Defence Forces[2] (Hooper, 1999:767–771)—were "killing a lot of people, destroying much property, and raping and looting" (*New York Times*, 1979), a claim with which the older people of Masaka who still remember those days would wholeheartedly agree.

One such person—a 56-year-old businessman whom I got to know well during the five years I lived in Masaka—told me of his experiences. "When the first bombs burst in town," he told me, "I was here. But I had to run away. First I went to my village, which is about eight miles from here, and then from there, I travelled and went to Kampala. Many people left; they abandoned the town. They went because they were scared of the war. But all our property was left here, so it was looted. Everything was taken. We were left with nothing, not even a mattress. It was very dangerous to stay in such a place. These Amin people were trying to hide among the civilians, so it was not advisable to keep around. We had to run away and hide somewhere. And when we came back, we found everything taken. The houses were unroofed, they took away the iron sheets, the doors, the windows; the town was just left naked. All these houses, these old houses, they have since been replaced or repaired. They were just firing on the houses. I remember a very big building, a hall, it was completely put down. Banks, commercial banks, those were the major ones; they were down. Plus some beautiful houses around Villa Maria road. When the Tanzanians entered here, they were seeing these beautiful houses and they thought they were ministers' houses. So people lost a lot. They lost a lot. I think I have never again experienced poverty like that."

The looting, murder, and rape inflicted upon Masaka during the 1979 invasion devastated the town and its surrounding rural areas. A *New York Times* report from one year later, in April 1980, explains how Masaka, formerly Uganda's third largest town, had been "all but leveled . . . Today about 6,000 residents remain among the rubble . . . Masaka District, once one of the most prosperous agricultural centers in Uganda, has pretty much returned to subsistence farming" (*New York Times*, 1980).

Among the rubble and poverty that remained throughout the district, the seeds of the world's first catastrophic community-wide AIDS epidemic had already been sown, a direct product of the rape and social disruption that had characterized the war. HIV and AIDS were as yet unknown, with the first reports of a hitherto unidentified "cellular-immune dysfunction related to a common exposure" found in five young homosexual men in Los Angeles not due for publication until June 1981 (CDC, 1981); but it is likely that the virus had been lurking at low levels for some time in Uganda, and that the very particular conditions brought about during and directly after the war facilitated its rapid spread through Rakai and Masaka at that moment (see Hooper, 1999:31–51).

Ironically, Idi Amin himself—a man with little formal education— seemed to have been aware that an unusual disease was being spread during the war of 1978–79. A local journalist in Masaka told me how, "in the closing stages of the war, Amin had spoken of how the *wakombozi* [the invading forces from Tanzania] are also spreading a dangerous type of gonorrhea. He said it is incurable, and its victim wastes away and loses all the hair."

This was confirmed by Dr. Wilson Carswell, a Scotsman who worked as a consultant surgeon at Kampala's Mulago Hospital between 1968 and 1987, and who led most of the first AIDS research in Uganda. He told me when we met at his London office that Amin had made what amounted to the world's first official proclamation about AIDS. "Whatever faults Amin had," he said, "he had a good rapport with his soldiers, and they had seen something change. He named this disease 'Good Hope,' because once you had it, good hope was all you had left."

Kasensero—Epicenter of a Pandemic

The fishing village of Kasensero lies just eight kilometers north of the border with Tanzania, and was subjected to heavy bombardment before being occupied by the 207th Battalion of the Tanzanian People's Defence Forces during the 1979 invasion (Hooper, 1999:769). However, this is not the village's main claim to fame. Rather, it is known as the epicenter of the world's first devastating, population-wide AIDS epidemic, a distinction brought about as a direct result of the invasion and subsequent chaos. Wilson Carswell visited Kasensero in the mid-1980s, when its population was being decimated by the first wave of AIDS deaths, and he told me that "although it's called a fishing village, it's really a trading outpost and entry port. Legal authorities call it smuggling. I think there's a bit of sex in some of the transactions, too."

I travelled there in order to speak with people who had experienced those early days of the epidemic, and to try to understand how they had perceived what was befalling their community. My guide for the day was a young local politician, 27 years old, and also, it emerged, an AIDS orphan herself. Her own story, while perhaps an extreme example, is illustrative of the profound extent to which AIDS has affected this corner of Uganda. "My father died in January 1984 when I was six," she told me as we set off down the bumpy road toward Kasensero, "and my mother died in December 1984, when I was seven." Her grandparents, she continued, had produced 18 children, of whom 17 were now dead. And from these 18 children, there had been born 73 grandchildren, of whom only 23 still lived. We passed by her grandparents' homestead on our way down to Lake Victoria, where she took me over to the banana plantation near the house, and pointed: "All of the places where there are flowers are where there are graves." I looked out over the banana plantation, blanketed in every direction with red, purple, and yellow flowers. Every flowerbed in this huge family graveyard covered the body of one of her parents, siblings, cousins, aunts, or uncles.

From the homestead, the landscape was wide open and empty as we drove down toward the lake, punctuated with the occasional escarpment that emerges out of the flat, swampy land. When we reached Kasensero, it was quietly busy, with fishermen fixing their nets on the beach and women cooking maize cobs over charcoal fires in the streets. We passed through alleyways lined with refuse and pools of murky water, which disappeared into the maze of flimsy-looking wooden shacks. Our first respondent was a man who had worked on some of the very first HIV prevention campaigns in the area during the late 1980s, and was held to be a local authority on the subject.

It started when the Tanzanian war happened [he told us].

People thought—it was rumored—that our soldiers had stolen some commodities from Tanzania. And because the Tanzanians were very good at charming,[3] people thought it was just one way of charming. The cause was those soldier-thieves. That was the first idea I had.

By the time Amin was driven out, he warned people: 'You people, take care! You are going to get a gonorrhea which takes off your hair. You will get bald heads! And this gonorrhea is from Tanzania.' And as time went on, more people got infected, and their private parts were being eaten up by the disease. Sometimes the intestines would come out. The skin turned to blue, and there were wounds and boils. Some of them had mental problems.

At first we were taking it as bewitchery from these Tanzanians. The hair getting off, fever, and they were emaciated. People would fear the victims, fear that the witchcraft was infectious, so there was a lot of stigma, even though they took it for granted that it was bewitchery. The emaciation was too much. You could see a young man looking very old. Diarrhea was too much. Some could take in food and it would pass out the same as when they ate it. It was a strange disease; it was a wasting disease. The word Slim was born here. At that time, people put on very tight clothes, for fashion. So from that, we got the word Slim. But nobody knew how it was transmitted.[4]

We passed by a fish-processing plant on the way to our next informant, who was working in the fisheries office where the daily catch is checked and counted. We sat in his small wooden office, and my guide introduced me, explaining my interest in the very beginning of the epidemic.

"There was a lady during the war," he began. "She was called Nantongo Rose. She started showing signs as she was moving around, looking for a safe place to avoid the fighting. When she came back here after the war, she was too weak. She had emaciated, and her skin had become very bright, and she lost her hair. The emaciation forced her to take it for granted that she was bewitched. She didn't have diarrhea, or vomiting, but she had fever. She tried to get treatment, but she deteriorated and died in 1980. She had been bedridden for eight months."

I asked him what he thought then had been the cause of her sickness. "As it was a new disease, a new problem, I also had an idea that it was witchcraft," he explained. "At first there were these young men, and they would go into Tanzania to buy things, as merchants. We thought that they had stolen things from Tanzania, and the Tanzanians bewitched them with terrible bewitching that could not be cured. Some said that they had stolen these *mukene* fish[5] and had been cursed as a result. It was something called *muteego*, which is the type of witchcraft which is meant to wipe out an entire family. They even went to witchdoctors in Tanzania to cure it, but they failed. There was never even any rumor that they had been cured. But people still went because they were desperate."

Two points stand out from what these informants told me. First, they both believed that witchcraft stood behind the events they were witnessing—there was no suggestion that the terrible new disease called Slim was sexually transmitted. Second, this witchcraft had its origin in Tanzania, and had been inflicted on the people of Kasensero as vengeance for theft. As often happens during epidemics, therefore, it was "the other" who was blamed for bringing the disease "to us" (see, for example, Evans [1995], with respect to cholera in nineteenth-century Europe; and Farmer [1993] with respect to AIDS in Haiti during the 1980s and early 1990s).

These are important points, epidemiologically speaking, since they provided no basis for undertaking any sort of effective prevention activities such as we would understand them today. These could include, for example, reducing one's number of sexual partners, or using condoms. Wilson Carswell had described to me how there was "a bit of sex in some of the transactions" at Kasensero, which was really a euphemism for the well-established network of sex workers who earned their living in the fishing village. That was the case in the early 1980s, and it remains so today. As my guide in Kasensero explained to me, "[L]adies target the season when there are many fish at the lake. They dress smartly. The fishermen say that they earn their money, and if they have money, they want to have the girls. And the girls then circulate around all the different landing sites."[6] A few minutes after she told me this, three young women in tight trousers appeared, walking down the main road, having just arrived in the village. "You see!" my guide laughed. "They have come for business!"

As will be discussed in Chapter 4, condoms were hardly available in Uganda until well into the 1990s. And as such, Kasensero in the early- and mid-1980s—with its heady mixture of previous military action and occupation, ongoing and extensive prostitution, and a highly mobile population—therefore acted as a powerful vector for transmitting HIV far and wide, both within Uganda and beyond.

Atypical Kaposi's Sarcoma—The First Scientific Evidence of AIDS

Although Kasensero is widely held to be the epicenter of the epidemic, similar events were unfolding, if on a slightly smaller scale, in other parts of Rakai and Masaka—all the places, in fact, where the 207th Brigade of the TPDF had passed through in 1979 (Hooper, 1999:769). For example, 84 cases of Slim had been registered in Masaka's Kitovu hospital during 1982 alone (Tibomanya, 1992). But because continuing war and deep insecurity remained the norm throughout this part of Uganda,[7] the expanding epidemic was taking place in almost complete isolation from the rest of the world. No doctor outside the area, and no scientist or policy maker anywhere, even knew that anything was amiss.

However, in December 1983, Anne Bayley—a British physician based at the University Teaching Hospital in Lusaka, Zambia—was appointed President of the Association of Surgeons in East Africa, an organization that each year brought together colleagues from six English-speaking countries throughout the region. At her inaugural lecture that month in Kampala, she described an atypical and particularly aggressive form of Kaposi's sarcoma (KS) that she had been encountering with increasing frequency over the previous 12 months back in Lusaka.[8] Unlike the KS that all the surgeons present at the meeting were familiar with, this variety attacked women as well as men, it presented centrally and not just peripherally, and, crucially, it did not respond well to treatment. Bayley reported that she had seen ten of the old-style KS patients that year, and they were all still alive; but she had also seen thirteen cases of this more aggressive variety over the same period, and eight were now dead (Bayley, 1984). She asked colleagues to look out for similar developments elsewhere in the region, noting that several patients with the new, aggressive KS had also tested positive for HTLV-III.[9]

Wilson Carswell was present at the conference, and he explained that although he took note of the issue, he asked himself how serious Anne Bayley's suggestion could really be. "Is this just an interesting footnote?" he wondered. "There are so many other problems in Africa."

Nonetheless, footnote or not, one of the striking things about the discussion that took place at the conference was that while Bayley was implicitly referring to AIDS, Carswell says that the word "AIDS" was never used. At that time, the disease was generally recognized to exist only in homosexual Western populations,[10] and, given that homosexuality is considered to be an abomination throughout much of Africa, the surgeons recognized the need for self-censorship. "You had to talk in terms of HTLV-III-related KS," Carswell explained, "or that it was aggressive KS, or that it may have been similar to the KS that has been described in the U.S."

But the issue intrigued Carswell, and, early in 1984, he was approached by a colleague who had also attended the surgeons' conference: Bob Downing, a virologist from the Public Health Laboratory Services in Porton Down, England. Downing wanted to test some Ugandan KS samples for HTLV-III, and Carswell agreed to assist, so he bled eleven KS patients at Mulago hospital and sent the samples to Porton Down for evaluation: nine of the eleven samples tested HTLV-III positive. Anne Bayley's findings from Zambia were thus corroborated, and, for the first time, "we had established that HTLV-III-related KS also existed in Uganda" (Bayley et al., 1985).

However, Carswell recognized that the very small sample size limited the epidemiological significance of his findings, so, in anticipation of a forthcoming conference at which he would be presenting, he went to the records for something more substantial:

> Imperial Cancer Research had set up in Kampala a databank on all the recorded cancers based on histology. Surgeons took a specimen and put it in a bottle with some formalin and a screw cap, and then put it in a specially prepared hollowed-out piece of wood, with a lid, and a label on it. All the histology from all the country went to the histology department at Makerere Medical School. And despite the fact that the record-keeping fell apart, in a monumental way [because of the civil war], this did not apply to this cancer registry. There was one little man there—he must have had obsessive-compulsive disorder!—who kept records. The world was falling apart, and he kept records! There was demographic data on the forms—name, age, tribe, place of residence. They were filed by year, all of 1980 was together, for example, and they were coded according to the International Classification of Disease, so it was fairly easy to flick through them.
>
> So I walked up to the cancer registry and said can I see the records. I went through the records between 1980, 81, 82, 83 and 84, because five years seemed a reasonable number. And it was pretty easy to decide based on the information supplied whether they were classic African Kaposi's, or whether they weren't: looking for not-middle-aged, or a woman, or if they were central nodes. If it was typical KS, the doctors would say this is KS, but if it was atypical, they'd say I don't know what it is. But then it would be classified as KS on histology. The histologist classified it. And on the basis of clinical history, then one was able to judge whether it was typical or atypical. And from about 1982 onwards, they were getting atypical KS. They didn't have it in 1980.

The presence of HTLV-III, as identified by Bob Downing, in combination with the increasing numbers of atypical KS cases shown in the Makerere histology records, provided a clear indication that AIDS had taken hold in Uganda. The scale of what was to follow could not possibly have been anticipated at that stage, but, in any event, the ongoing war stifled any attempt to control the nascent epidemic at the time, or even to conduct any sort of surveillance. Throughout 1984, in the central and western parts of the country, Yoweri Museveni's rebel National Resistance Army was battling with President Milton Obote's troops, who in turn were supported by gunners from North Korea. The rural population was being terrorized, tens of thousands of people had been displaced from their homes, and a few cases of a strange new disease were of little interest to a government that faced the much more urgent and immediate concern of fighting a war.

Reports from Rakai and Confusion over Etiology

There may have been little official interest in the phenomenon, but the story did not, of course, disappear. In November 1984, Dr. Anthony Lwegaba was serving as the first District Medical Officer in the newly created Rakai district (Rakai had formerly been part of Masaka district), and he sent a report to the Ministry of Health detailing the new condition. The symptoms he described in the report went from general malaise and sporadic fever to diarrhea, loss of weight and color, and then skin rashes and a dry cough. "In view of the fact," he concluded, "that all long standing diseases inevitably cause wasting or body weight loss—a cardinal sign in Slim—then Slim might not be one disease but a collection of diseases" (Lwegaba, 1984; cited in Iliffe, 1998:222). AIDS was mentioned in the piece, though only as one of several possible causes of Slim.

No immediate action was taken by the Ministry as a result of the report. The next month, at the end of December, the first public report of AIDS was published in a Kampala-based newspaper called *The Star*. With the dramatic headline "Mysterious Disease Kills 100 People in Rakai," the report is worth repeating in full here—both for what it says as well as for what it does not say.

> A strange killer disease has struck the District of Rakai in South Uganda, killing at least 100 people in ten months. The victims of the disease, locally called 'SLIM,' are youths aged between 15 to 36 years. The worst hit area is Kyebe-Kannebulemu sub-county. Hardly a fortnight passes without a death of one or more young men or women. Mourning is everywhere and several people I met wear dejected faces, carry heavy hearts and are living in great fear.
>
> The disease has so far not responded to any treatment. All patients taken to various hospitals have died. Investigations I made here indicated that the disease has been prevalent in the district for over a year now. The disease,

which started at Kyebe-Kannebulemu, has now spread to Kyotera Township and Kooki.

A common characteristic about this disease is that all victims have at one time or another been associated with the lucrative border trade between Uganda and Tanzania. Once one has contracted it, one experiences intermittent fits of vomiting, diarrhea, preceded and accompanied by fever, high temperatures and profuse perspiration. Despite treatment of whatever nature, the condition persists. Gradually, the victim loses weight and progressively gets so emaciated that within a fortnight or month, he is reduced to mere skin-on-bones with eyes nakedly sticking out of fleshless sockets. The sick young person miserably and desperately awaits the imminent and inevitable end—death. Although several people have consulted professional doctors, all people I talked to said they have completely failed to get a remedy for this killer disease.

In the last six months alone, more than 40 people have died. Some families have lost more than one of their youth. To mention but a few of those families, Laurio Nnoba of Kinyiga village lost two twin sons aged 32 and another son following them. Ferdinand Kagezi of Balole village has lost two sons and a daughter-in-law; Karko Kasujju of Gwanda village has lost two sons, and recently three cases, namely Muluba, Bukenya and Nsamba were reportedly taken to Mulago Hospital, Kampala.

The people I interviewed appealed to the government, especially the Ministry of Health, to immediately embark on a plan to save the families of Rakai District.

(*Star*, 1984)

Notable in this piece is the fact that no mention is made of AIDS, of the disease being sexually transmitted, or of witchcraft. The only attempt to suggest an etiology, or cause, for the condition was the point that "all victims have at one time or another been associated with the lucrative border trade between Uganda and Tanzania."

According to several people I interviewed, this piece was widely read, and it raised considerable concern: a number of doctors connected to the Ministry of Health now had firm suspicions that this condition was AIDS. Still, some time passed before any action was taken. Dr. David Serwadda, then a Senior House Officer at Mulago Hospital and now Dean of the Makerere University School of Public Health in Kampala, explained that after reading the Lwegaba report and then the *Star* article, "the Minister of Health quickly convened a meeting in Mulago to discuss the situation. Dr. M [a senior government epidemiologist] attended, and I remember telling him that we know what's going on in Rakai. We already knew that this disease was associated with HTLV-III. In April 1984, I had seen a Time magazine article in which Gallo had linked AIDS with HTLV-III.[11] Soon after, we started sending samples for testing via Carswell: we took off blood and sent it to Porton Down. I remember in July 1984 receiving an airmail letter in the post saying that one set of our samples had tested HTLV-III positive. So by the time the *Star* report came out, we had a fair collection of samples, and I said to M, I think this is AIDS. He dismissed it, because it was seen as a disease of white homosexual males."

An investigative team was finally sent by the Ministry of Health down to Rakai in February 1985, and their report concluded that the Slim-related deaths there were due to unsanitary conditions. Wilson Carswell believes that the lead author of the report, Professor B, genuinely felt that this outbreak was caused by typhoid, and that the report did not constitute a high-level whitewash: "He just said they were dirty people, and they should dig more latrines." As with Doctor M's dismissal of the hypothesis, the possibility of this disease being AIDS apparently lay outside Professor B's mental framework at the time. "AIDS was seen by the authorities as a homosexual disease," explained Carswell, "so, ipso facto, AIDS could not exist in Uganda."[12]

This was a common refrain of the time, and it was not restricted to Uganda. A physician who went on to hold a senior position with UNAIDS in Geneva was struggling with similar frustrations over etiology, but in relation to the epidemic in Kinshasa, the capital city of what was then Zaire. He told me that he had his "aha experience" about AIDS when he and other colleagues were invited by the Zairian government to conduct an exploratory study on the new condition in October 1983. He explained how he was shocked to see people "my own age" lying there. "I thought this is something different. Either this is a short-lived outbreak, or we're in deep trouble." He had been around in Zaire long enough to know "how people behave" sexually, he said, so the possibility of its being AIDS was present in his mind. The initial question for him, therefore, was, "Is this the same thing that's going on as what's happening with the white gay men?" He noticed striking differences to the gay epidemic, such as the relative youth of those who were sick in Kinshasa, as well as the almost equal ratio of men and women. But he was also able to make a crucial mental leap, and, as he told me, to ask, "Why would a virus care about the sexual orientation of its host?"

The conclusion of his study was clear, as was the explicit use of the word "AIDS": "Thirty eight patients with the acquired immunodeficiency syndrome (AIDS) were identified in Kinshasa, Zaire, during a three week period in 1983 . . . The findings of this study strongly argue that the situation in central Africa represents a new epidemiological setting for this worldwide disease—that of significant transmission in a large hetero-sexual population" (Piot et al., 1984:65–66). Nonetheless, this paper faced fierce opposition during the peer review process prior to publication: the editorial panel of the *New England Journal of Medicine*, to which it was first sent, could not accept the suggestion that AIDS was spread heterosexually, and it was rejected (Garrett, 1994:347). A resubmission to the *Lancet* finally concluded in publication.

The difficulty in accepting the heterosexual nature of AIDS was therefore by no means restricted to government bureaucrats in Kampala: some high-level international scientists felt the same way. But since there was virtually no contact or collaboration between the small handful of AIDS researchers who were active in Africa at that time and who could see what was going on, a substantive challenge to this critical misconception was not mounted. These researchers included the group in Kinshasa (called Project SIDA); another collaboration in Kigali, Rwanda, who had also explicitly used the word "AIDS" in relation to what they were finding in a heterosexual population (van de Perre, 1984); Anne Bayley in Zambia; and Carswell with his colleagues in Kampala, who were obliged to talk publicly in terms of HTLV-III-related KS, or Slim. As Carswell himself laments, "[I]n Africa, Francophones and Anglophones don't speak," so an early opportunity to join forces against the burgeoning epidemic was lost.

A Trip to Masaka—Recognition and Denial

Dr. Carswell's first opportunity to investigate the issue for himself at the heart of the Ugandan epidemic arose in June 1985, around the time of that year's final clinical examination for Makerere University's medical undergraduates.

"In order to be correct, the surgery exam needed an external auditor. At that time, with the war on, it was a bit like Iraq: hands up, who wants to be an external examiner in Uganda? We couldn't get anybody from the U.K., so they got Anne Bayley instead—she was a professor in Lusaka, she'd been President of the Association of Surgeons, she was well respected. And we did the exams, and then I said let's go down and see about this. Let's go down to Rakai." Anne Bayley had been the surgeon who had called attention in December 1983 to the atypical KS she was seeing in Zambia, so she was clearly an appropriately qualified colleague for an investigative field trip such as this. With her assent, Carswell assembled a team of medics from Kampala,[13] and they set off to Rakai:

> We went down on the Saturday morning in our orange Kombi van, down to Kalisizo [the first town encountered in Rakai district when driving from Masaka or Kampala], and there were half a dozen patients in the hospital there, and two of them had Slim. We left the physicians to examine them and take their histories and so on, and then Anne Bayley and myself had nothing

to do, being redundant surgeons, so we went into the nearest slum town. We started talking to the guys, and said we were interested in Slim, because that was what we'd heard it was called, and we asked have you seen any? "Yeah, we've seen a couple." And we walked into the more under-developed part of the town, and we found a couple of people with Slim. So we put them in the Kombi and took them back to Kalisizo, and the physicians examined them. Took their stools, and we bled them, and then we took them back.

And then this was really just a stopover, and we really wanted to go to the fishing village [Kasensero], and do the proper study that wasn't done earlier [by the Ministry of Health investigative team four months previously]. So we said, we'll stay in Masaka overnight, and then we'll go to the village at the crack of dawn, get there about seven or seven thirty, work till about four, and then take two hours to get back to Kampala before dark. Don't go out after dark, you get shot—there's a war on! But that evening, we went into Masaka hospital itself, because the Medical Superintendent had been a student of mine, and I said we're looking for Slim, and he said, "yeah, we've got a case." Well, it's nearly dark now, so we decided to come back first thing in the morning, and have a look. So eight o'clock Sunday morning, good light, no doctors, no nurses, lots of patients, and lots of relatives. So what do surgeons do when they're stuck? They do a ward round. So we did a quick ward round. Just the two of us, Anne and me. Serwadda and the others were looking at this one patient. We did this quick ward round, you go round the ward and see what the pattern is, what's happening, and I think there were 90-odd people in the hospital, and we thought 29 of them might have Slim. So we were now on Plan B—we scrapped the fishing village in Rakai, and we spent the whole day just weighing and measuring and watching and bleeding and taking stools in Masaka.[14]

That was the first week in June, and by the end of June, there was yet another East African surgeons meeting, this time in Blantyre, and basically I presented this paper there. At that time, the [London-based] *Daily Telegraph* was running a campaign for Virginia Slim cigarettes: "Slim is a four-letter word meaning elegance." In English. But it also meant something else in south-west Uganda. They said they were slimming to death. They said, "we have Slim."

In addition to the Blantyre presentation, the outcome of this trip to Rakai and Masaka was a groundbreaking article in the *Lancet*, the first publication in the scientific literature to describe clinical cases of AIDS in Uganda,[15] and the first to describe an epidemic of AIDS in a general rural population anywhere in the world. It also revealed that every one of the 29 patients bled in Masaka hospital had tested seropositive for HTLV-III (Serwadda et al., 1985:851), the key serological marker for AIDS among homosexual men in Western countries. However, in spite of this, the piece concluded that "although Slim disease resembles AIDS in many ways, it seems to be a new entity" (ibid., 850). The apparent basis for this distinction was that "although many of the features of Slim disease satisfy the criteria for AIDS," Slim is characterized by "extreme weight loss and diarrhea" (ibid., 851)—notwithstanding the fact that these two symptoms were also striking many AIDS patients in the West. In other words, the official, public interpretation of what they had seen was not in accordance with what at least some of them privately believed to be the case. I asked Wilson Carswell why this was.

> Oh, that was political. Self-censorship [he explained]. I think unless we'd put it in, it wouldn't have got published [because the paper first had to be cleared by the Ugandan authorities]. You have to read between the lines on these things, and use obscure language that only a social scientist would understand! I mean, you can say what you like, but the great thing about Uganda during the time of the dictators—Amin and Obote—was that when you published something, between the lines there was always a white space. And as long as there's space between the lines, you can read between them. Such things happened quite often. I remember the leader of a rebellion came in [to his Mulago Hospital operating theatre] with two pistol shots to his epigastrium. He died. And Amin came in to inspect the body, so he could make sure that the chap was dead. Then I had to write a post mortem report, indicating suicide, even if it's pretty difficult to give yourself two pistol wounds! So I was adept at writing things like that.
>
> Anyway, this was for publication. What did we say to the Ministry? We said, you've got AIDS in this country. And there's lots of it, clinical cases. And in apparently healthy people. The people with Slim, they're beyond, you know, it's too late. But the important thing is these healthy people.

I asked the same question to David Serwadda, who was the first author on the paper, and who had also been on the Masaka trip: Why did you not *say* that you had seen AIDS in Masaka, as this could have had important implications for prevention and control strategies? He told me he did not remember the particular wording they had used, but he suggested that "it may have been hard for people to believe that this disease was the same as the one striking white male homosexuals. People would have wondered how it could have come so fast to Rakai and Masaka." Nonetheless, regardless of what the paper did or did not say—or of what was or was not written between the lines—Serwadda was disappointed by the response from the authorities within the Ministry, even though he, like Carswell, worked behind the scenes to raise awareness about the problem.

"When the *Lancet* paper came out in October 1985," he explained, "it was widely publicized in the news outlets—though not locally—but nobody ever called me to ask about its implications. I had to be proactive, distributing it in the Ministry. There's a culture within the Ministry of not reading: things just drop on people's desks. So there wasn't a wide enthusiasm. Mixed feelings, at best. It's difficult to know whether the lack of interest was because people had other things on their minds. Remember this was the time of Obote 2 and Okello,[16] and there was very difficult instability. A lot of struggle. And the priorities were very different."

The priorities in the Ministry of Health may have been very different, but it was clear that the data described in this paper represented just the tip of a large iceberg, and that more research was needed in order to determine what action would be most appropriate. The need for urgent action had been made clear to Carswell by the very people who were suffering from AIDS. "We'd listened to the people in Kalisizo and Masaka," he recalled. "They'd said, 'what are you going to do for us? We're dying!'"

Carswell and the virologist Bob Downing therefore drew up a proposal for a three-year epidemiological study to be conducted in Rakai, which was intended primarily to identify risk groups. They presented it to the Ministry of Health's Disease Surveillance Sub-Committee (DSSC) in order to obtain approval prior to the request for funding, but the response was not positive. The very same Professor B who, one year previously, had determined that the Slim epidemic in Rakai was typhoid wrote to the subcommittee. According to Carswell's notes from the time, the letter stated that "it is undesirable to overplay the danger of AIDS, since this could easily divert attention from other causes of morbidity, and bring about unwanted anxiety and hysteria."

I asked Carswell why he thought the proposal evoked such a response from Professor B. "I think he felt it genuinely [that the danger of AIDS should not be overplayed]." he explained. "But I also think he was irritated by the fact that we were these bloody foreigners coming in and doing virology studies." Consequently, "the DSSC was adamant that the heterosexual mode of transmission should not be stressed in a statement on health education." Thus the study proposal for Rakai was rejected, and a period of firm official denial about AIDS had taken root in Uganda. Meanwhile, a limited public information campaign about AIDS was instigated by the Ministry of Health, based around the rather ambiguous message "Love Carefully." In the absence of any further explanation, it was difficult for people to know how they should act on this.

But in mitigation to those who did not, or could not believe what was going on, there had been revelations that some of the earliest tests for HTLV-III had significantly overestimated prevalence rates by producing what was known as sticky serum.[17] The most notorious of these cases was published in the prestigious journal *Science* by a team led by Carl Saxinger from the U.S.-based National Cancer Institute. The piece reported that 50 out of 75 children from the West Nile region of Uganda had tested HTLV-III-positive, and it concluded that HTLV-III may have been "existing in a population acclimated to its presence" (Saxinger et al., 1985:1036). This effectively meant that HTLV-III was harmless, and that something else was responsible for AIDS. The suggestion was lent considerable weight because one of the paper's coauthors was Robert Gallo, one of two powerful men who had claimed to be the discoverer of the virus in the first place.

The sticky serum phenomenon precipitated one of innumerable controversial theories that have emerged about AIDS over the course of the epidemic. Although the very high prevalence rates reported were found relatively quickly to be an artifact of a particular virological testing technique rather than an indication of actual events on the ground, it brought about serious problems at the time. Carswell recalled that this paper "caused us headaches from the moment it was published," a view reflected by a Belgian scientist who was working on AIDS in Rwanda during the mid-1980s. Even when it became clear that the findings from this particular study were wildly misleading, "[Saxinger] never retracted his research," the Belgian told me, "or held a press conference to say his data was incorrect and explain why, and as a result it made our work very difficult. It was very damaging. You could go to a Minister with a suggestion, and he would just point to this study and say, 'you see, it's all untrue. We know that now.'" This study provided a perfect, ready-made justification for officialdom to sit on its hands: scientists themselves had actively facilitated AIDS denial.

Sticky serum data notwithstanding, the available evidence pointed to a very severe epidemic in Uganda, far more so than in any other African country for which information was available. The annual incidence of AIDS in Kinshasa had been pegged, albeit conservatively, at 17 per 100,000, meaning that an estimated 0.017 percent of the population would be expected to fall sick with AIDS each year (Piot et al., 1984); while the incidence in Kigali, Rwanda, was estimated at 80 per 100,000, equivalent to 0.08 percent per year (Van de Perre et al., 1984).[18] Meanwhile, a group of healthy controls in a Zambian study had shown HTLV-III prevalence rates of 2 percent; and an equivalent group of healthy controls in Uganda showed 20 percent prevalence (Bayley et al., 1985). The scale of what was happening in Uganda therefore appeared to be an order of magnitude greater than anything being seen anywhere else, and with the potential for heterosexual transmission of HTLV-III now well established in African populations (Clumeck et al., 1985; Kreiss et al., 1986), restricting public information to a limited and opaque "Love Carefully" message was likely only to exacerbate the situation.

By now, a major crisis was therefore in the making. At the end of 1985, Carswell says that AIDS had become the second most common cause of admission to the medical wards at Mulago Hospital, and, on the basis of clinical manifestations, was the most common cause of death. Furthermore, the backdrop to all this, as described in his unpublished memoirs, was certainly not conducive to mounting an effective response to AIDS:

> At this time shooting was heard nearly every night, and at some times a quarter of the patients in the surgical wards were suffering from gunshot wounds. The south-west of the country [Masaka and Rakai] was cut off from the capital. Some Ugandan doctors had fled the country and others were trying to leave. Morale could not have been lower. Outside bodies were not interested in Uganda's problems, least of all in AIDS. Those of us who were interested were left to our own devices. Despite this depressing background we felt that a lot had been achieved with very little resources. Thanks to our links with PHLS [the Public Health Laboratory Service in Porton Down, England], we were able to confirm a number of cases, and it was increasingly obvious to all of us still involved that we were at the start of a major epidemic of AIDS.
>
> (Carswell, 1987: unpublished memoirs)

Carswell had conducted a study in October 1985, which, through his links with PHLS, had shown that 10 out of a sample of 103 women attending Mulago hospital's antenatal clinic were infected with HTLV-III (Carswell, personal communication). Since pregnant women provide a fair reflection of healthy young adults in society as a whole, surgery itself was now becoming a major risk factor for infection. With characteristic understatement, Carswell described how, as a surgeon, the high rates of HTLV-III infection in the general population "made one more reluctant to give blood" to a patient on the operating table. After all, if one in ten of all pregnant women was carrying the virus, what proportion of blood donors was also infected?

The Tide Turns: Official Acceptance of AIDS, and the Establishment of the National AIDS Control Programme

As a senior consultant surgeon at Mulago hospital, Carswell had to deal with three Ministers of Health who worked for three different Presidents, one after the other: Minister Nkwasibwe under Obote, Minister Obonyo under Okello, and Minister Rugunda under Museveni. "I had entry to the big shots because they'd known me when they were students. The first two didn't last long, but I told them that this was AIDS. They weren't very interested. Rugunda had been a student of mine too. He was quite interested, but he had other things on his plate. It was difficult to convince the politicians."

I asked him why he thought this was. "Perhaps it was a matter of poor presentation of the available data," he replied. "They simply couldn't conceive that if 30 out of 100 people were infected but healthy, that they would die. They just couldn't visualize it."

It took nothing less than a presidential leap of imagination to bring about the first steps toward establishing serious AIDS control measures in the country. Yoweri Museveni's rebel army had entered Kampala on 26 January 1986, bringing to an end Uganda's long civil war, and although Uganda's epidemic was clearly more advanced than those in neighboring Zaire and Rwanda, the country's response was lagging seriously behind.

In his unpublished memoirs, Carswell describes a meeting with the new President that he and several colleagues attended in September 1986:

> When we arrived at the appointed time to see the President, he was just finishing a solitary lunch, served on modest plastic plates. The meeting opened with the President asking us how many of us were working full time on AIDS, as it was a serious problem. The answer was that none of us was full time. Museveni said that he had had many queries about AIDS from worried individuals as he had travelled around the country. The tenor of his questions was to seek information about AIDS in general and to find out what was being done about it. He said he knew that the disease was now a problem in the south-west, and seemed aware of how it could be contained. Like many others, he queried the role of mosquitoes in transmitting the AIDS virus. He also suggested that mothers—who prepared local medicines by chewing ingredients, usually leaves and similar materials, before giving it to their children—might pass it to them that way. S[19] was very proud of the Love Carefully pamphlet which had been produced at his instigation, and he wanted to present a bundle to the President. Museveni, however, was loathe to accept them and did not even undo the bundle. He said that the leaflets would not be of much use, as most people in the country could not read, and of those who could, not all could read English, the only language the pamphlet was printed in. In this he showed more insight than many of his experts.
>
> (Carswell, 1987: unpublished memoirs)

There was unanimous agreement among those of my respondents who were engaged at this time about the critical role played by the new President. One emphasized Museveni's thirst for knowledge. He told me that on one occasion in 1986, he had given a presentation to the Cabinet about a study he had conducted at a truck stop in Rakai, and he joked how afterwards the President had "quizzed [him] like hell" about his findings.

David Serwadda pointed out that Museveni had been well aware of AIDS before he came to power: "Museveni had heard of it. He had an awareness, so that when he came in he was very open about it. When he was [fighting] in the bush, he had listened to the BBC, and they were touching on the published papers [from the U.S. as well as his own 1985 *Lancet* article]. But he also likes to get information through conversation. When we met with him, he was able to grasp the way we described HIV and the immune system, because he could relate it to a military context."

A senior virologist working in Entebbe told a similar story of presidential engagement in the issue: "The major influence was HE [His Excellency the President]. We had a meeting at State House, and I remember him saying 'we have an enemy, and we're going to fight that enemy.' It was easy to make the military link."

But this military link did not stop with the simple parallel between the "battle" between HIV and an individual's immune system; or indeed between the country's responding to the "invading" virus. It should be remembered that Museveni came to power as the leader of a rebel army, and, as he recalled in a BBC interview, his concern for AIDS was at least partially triggered by the high infection rates among the very soldiers he was relying on to keep him in power.

"We had to send sixty soldiers to Cuba for military training. Fortunately for the Cubans, they were already testing the blood status of people while here we had not. In fact, there were only two machines in the whole of Uganda at that time. Now when they tested our sixty soldiers they found that eighteen out of the sixty had the virus. And when I was in the [Non-Aligned Movement] meeting in Harare—1986—Dr. Fidel Castro told me of this . . . I had heard a little bit about AIDS one year before but this one sprung me into action" (Museveni, 2003).

Under the difficult circumstances of the time, the process of springing into action took place reasonably quickly. By October 1986, the new Ugandan government had established the National Committee for the Prevention and Control of AIDS, which subsequently evolved into the National AIDS Control Programme (ACP). Carswell describes the opening ceremony thus:

> They had a gold-printed invitation, and the man in charge was Batwala [Deputy Minster of Health], a well-connected gynecologist. The chief guest was the Save the Children Fund, because WHO was effectively not present, mentally or physically or spiritually, in Uganda. And Batwala was quoting data that he *knew* wasn't correct. He said that AIDS isn't really a big problem in this country, because in the whole of Africa up to today, there are only

440 cases—which was what WHO had said. But at that time, we were getting 100 cases a month in Kampala alone, confirmed cases, and they were dying. So to mention WHO was disingenuous.

The now-fabled Ugandan openness about AIDS had therefore not yet quite flowered, and not all the guests held what Carswell considered to be helpful views either. "I was sitting there with the head of Save the Children at that time, and she said what would you like most, and I said I'd like a container of condoms. And she said, well, we can't have that! Because although she was Save the Children, she was also from an Irish Catholic background, and that was a bit extreme."

But a significant start had been made nonetheless, not least through the introduction at the opening ceremony of an important concept that was to become one of the mainstays of Uganda's early struggle against HIV: "Zero-grazing," an agricultural term that is immediately understood by anyone in this largely agrarian society. Zero-grazing refers to feeding one's livestock exclusively within the paddock, but the humorous double meaning that applies to HIV prevention maintains that one grazes, sexually speaking, also within the paddock. The paddock can include an exclusive, monogamous relationship, or a closed polygamous circle of a husband with two or more wives.

In addition, the establishment of the ACP gave credibility and support to Carswell's ongoing efforts to set up a safe blood transfusion system. He explained how, initially, "we in the British Residents' Association had raised £5,000 to send a nun to the U.K. for training in testing, and we set up a basic lab" in Nsambya Hospital in Kampala. This program had already started operating in June 1986, and it had constituted the very first substantive control measure against HIV taken in the country. But it was clearly insufficient to the task, so Carswell looked further afield for funds. Before long, "we got money from the EEC [European Economic Community]. When we first approached them, we said it's an emergency, and they replied that it would take three months to get the funding through. So then we said, well, actually it's a disaster. And they said, OK, if it's a disaster, you can have the money immediately."

The result was that Kitovu hospital, the largest health facility serving Rakai and Masaka districts, was able to start screening its blood supply in January 1987. This was not a moment too soon—Carswell's own data, collected between May 1986 and March 1987, showed that 15 percent of male donors and 21 percent of female donors were carrying the recently renamed virus, HIV (Carswell, 1987). In other words, roughly one in every six of all patients who received a blood transfusion was being simultaneously infected with HIV.

Discussion

The process of establishing the first AIDS control policy in Uganda—represented by the establishment of the country's ACP—can be broadly characterized as two streams flowing against each other: one that included those people who were working toward this goal, and one including those who, actively or not, were opposing it. By providing a social history of events, this chapter has clarified the nature of these respective streams, and shown why, until 1986, the opposing stream was the stronger of the two.

One of the overriding points here is the fact that AIDS was, throughout the early 1980s, still a disease "under construction." This meant that there was no generally accepted definition of what it was—at international, national, or local level—and no widely accepted understanding of its implications. The fact that it took a great deal of negotiation in order for the concepts of "AIDS" and "HIV" to be fixed—as illustrated by the sticky serum controversy, as well as by the disagreement over nomenclature between Luc Montagnier and Robert Gallo—helps to explain some of the delays in setting up a response. After all, it is hard to mount effective control measures if there remains real uncertainty even among scientists about what it is that actually needs controlling.

Furthermore, within Uganda, linking the syndrome that was affecting gay communities in Western countries with the horror simultaneously striking heterosexual populations in Rakai, Masaka, and Kampala was by no means straightforward. Apart from the fact that the ongoing war made it very difficult for the authorities in Kampala to establish what was actually going on outside the capital, AIDS as a disease description simply did not fit the condition they were hearing about or seeing. They could not grasp the fact that AIDS could also be a heterosexually transmitted condition, so diagnosing it as typhoid—which fitted into the tropical disease paradigm that they were familiar with—was inherently more convincing. As the father of modern experimental medicine, Claude Bernard, noted in 1865, "[T]hat which we know is the greatest obstacle to learning that which we do not know" (cited in Grmek, 1990:71). It takes an unusual mind to break out from "that which we know," and to move into uncharted intellectual waters. Thus the imagined epidemic of many of the national level actors at that stage, limited by what they *thought* they knew, is an important explanatory factor for the early difficulties in accepting the situation and establishing a policy response.

There were, however, also those who sensed that this new disease could in fact be AIDS, but who nonetheless felt that it would be best if such views were downplayed—for the country as a whole, and also, perhaps, for themselves personally. While these people may have established an intellectual understanding of events, they still faced an emotional barrier to acceptance: a profound and quite understandable discomfort with the fact that a fearsome disease was now on the rampage, one that could strike them and their families down. If they could somehow convince themselves that the scale of events was smaller than it really was—if they could deny what was happening—then they could believe that they were safe, and that life would go on as normal. There are clear historical precedents for such denial during a public health emergency. The following words, written in 1833 during a cholera outbreak in Amsterdam, could—simply by switching the word "cholera" for the word "AIDS"—equally have been written in Uganda 150 years later: "When cholera first breaks out, many a fear-ridden individual will perhaps unjustifiably be frightened of already having contracted the disease, and it is advisable that these people not be alarmed by exaggerated figures regarding the numbers of patients" (Brunt and Ronden, 1991:87). Public officials have in the past played down the scale of a major epidemic both to keep the public from panicking, and also, I would argue, to keep themselves from panicking.

There were two or three possible turning points that could have hastened the process of establishing the national ACP: the report from Rakai by Dr. Lwegaba in November 1984, for example; the publication of the *Star* article in December the same year; and the official investigation to Rakai in February 1985. But, for the reasons just given, the forces of opposition at the national level could not, intellectually or emotionally, accept the unacceptable fact that AIDS had already taken hold in Uganda on a large scale. Through this, these possible turning points were missed.

While the imagined epidemic of many people working at the national level inhibited early efforts to control AIDS, the people at the local level, from Rakai and Masaka, continued to suffer and die. These were the people who had ironically named the disease Slim; who believed that this terrible wasting condition must have been the product of powerful Tanzanian witchcraft that they were unable to counter; and who were cut off from the rest of the world by war as they were decimated. A defenseless, alienated, and utterly vulnerable population, their epidemic was not only imagined, it was also *lived*. Wilson Carswell described how they had pleaded with him: "We'd listened to the people in Kalisizo and Masaka. They'd said, 'what are you going to do for us? We're dying!'" But with no support at all coming in from the outside—thanks both to the war and to the national-level forces of opposition described above—they were the ultimate victims of these events. There were a number of influences that may have helped eventually to bring about a policy response to AIDS, but the people whose communities were dying cannot be counted among them.

One of the most important of the forces working toward the estab-lishment of national AIDS control measures was the research activity undertaken in Uganda by Wilson Carswell, David Serwadda, and their colleagues. The role of research at the start of an epidemic should ideally aim to provide the most basic facts, first of all by presenting convincing evidence that an epidemic is actually taking place. With this established, researchers need then to take an active role during the phase in which explanatory models for the epidemic are being developed, by investigating what the disease actually *is*, as well as the nature of the pathogenic agent that causes it. They then need to ascertain the means by which this agent is spread. When this epidemiological understanding has been established, it is possible then to assess who is likely to be at risk, through which activi-ties, and what can be done to reduce that risk (Kager, 1998).

A few such epidemiological and clinical papers were published about AIDS in Uganda, but there was nonetheless a clear divide between what was spoken and written publicly and what was said in private. Political constraints obliged the researchers publicly to couch their findings in terms that required readers to read between the lines, a practice not nor-mally associated with scientific writing. Meanwhile, they worked hard behind the scenes to convince the politicians that this was in fact AIDS, and that something had to be done.

These behind-the-scenes activities are an important theme. David Serwadda sees the impact of the research—in its most formal sense, that of actual publications—as being relatively limited: "Between 1984—when we could actually link HTLV-III to AIDS—and 1987 or 1988, there may have been at best four or five published articles, as well as maybe a few conference abstracts. Frankly, I have reservations that any of these papers changed policy. To me the early policy changes were purely influenced by the political leadership. When Museveni came in, a lot changed."

The reason for Museveni's openness on the topic appears to be, at least in part, the fact that his own imagined AIDS epidemic had been brought alive during the war. Although the chaos that followed it both sowed the seeds and fertilized the early epidemic, it also, ironically, played a role in creating conditions for establishing the first control measures. Museveni had fought his way to power through Rakai and Masaka dis-tricts (Museveni, 1997:167–168), so he had seen with his own eyes how people were suffering. He had also travelled through the country dur-ing his first months in office, listening to people's questions and worries about the growing epidemic. Furthermore, as a guerrilla leader while still in the bush, he had listened to the BBC World Service on a short-wave radio in order to stay informed about political developments relating to the war he was fighting, and in so doing he also learned about the 1985

Serwadda-Carswell Masaka study. Thus, when he found himself in State House, he knew whom to talk to about AIDS. His decision to establish the national ACP in 1986 was therefore influenced not by the journal articles per se, but by information he took from the discussions he held with those who had published them. The publications were not important in their own right, not least because hardly anyone in Uganda had access to them. Rather, they were important because they gave authority to the few people who were in a position to speak to the one person who mattered: Museveni himself, who happened to have an open mind on the subject.

But research was by no means the only influence on Museveni. Putzel (2004:26) has described the "incentive structure" that his government faced, arguing that "overall, [Uganda] had little to lose and everything to gain by taking early action on HIV/AIDS." Uganda had no foreign invest-ment at that stage to speak of, and certainly no tourist industry, which meant that there was nothing to scare away by admitting to the presence of AIDS in the country. By contrast, the authorities in neighboring Kenya feared a mass exodus of investors and tourists if they followed a similar path, and this contributed to a long delay in making any major statement on the subject. President Daniel arap Moi finally declared AIDS to be a national emergency in 1999, by when Museveni's early decision to open up to foreign assistance to help fight AIDS had already brought an estimated $180 million into the country (Hogle et al., 2002:11).

One further factor contributed significantly to Museveni's decision. As a military man, he naturally respects men from similar backgrounds. Thus he took very seriously the warning that Fidel Castro gave him in 1986 about the level of HIV infection among his troops. If the well-being of Museveni's army was threatened, his own hold on power could be, too. In this respect, it was fortuitous that Ugandan troops had been sent to Cuba for training, a country that was then renowned for its uncompro-mising public health approach to AIDS control. The private meeting in Harare at which Castro informed Museveni of the problem had enormous long-term national significance for Uganda, and it is a prime example of how the multilevel linkages referred to in Chapter 2 can influence policy: two national heads of state meeting at an international conference, with one convincing the other of the need to address a microscopic, infectious pathogen that was wreaking havoc in the bodies of some of the most mobile people in his country.

Reviewing the events that eventually led to the formation of Uganda's national ACP, one may be struck by the apparent intransigence of those actors who opposed this policy, as well as by the frustration felt by those who were working toward it. There was little or no sense of urgency in many quarters, and indeed some people were actively obstructive. But while this may be the case, it is also important to put these points into a wider perspective. Given the difficult conditions of war, of uncertainty at all levels about what AIDS actually was, and of the reticence felt by Uganda's neighbors to concede that they had an AIDS problem, it is remarkable how quickly the country's first AIDS control policy came into being.

4

Working on a Hunch: A History of HIV Prevention in Uganda

Introduction

Sitting in his Geneva office, a senior UNAIDS executive explained how he saw the role of evidence in the formulation of HIV prevention policy. "There is a spectrum," he said, "from having no data—in which case you do whatever you want, based on your hunch or on political expediency—to evidence-based decision making. And in the area of behavioral HIV prevention, there's very little evidence, so there's a move from [the principle of] evidence-based decision making back to value-based decision making."

These were broad-brush comments, intended to encapsulate the wider process of HIV prevention policy making in countries across the globe. In many respects, they also capture much of what has happened in Uganda since HIV prevention measures were initiated in the country in 1986. But, while there has indeed been very little evidence to guide prevention policy, and while much of the decision making process has indeed been value-based, the situation in Uganda has actually been rather more nuanced and complicated than this generic description suggests.

This is the topic of the present chapter, which charts the evolving relationship between HIV prevention research, policy, and practice, from 1986—when President Museveni launched the national AIDS Control Programme (ACP)—up until 2005. An important backdrop to the material presented is the major change that has taken place over the past decade or so in the rhetoric associated with health policy formulation. As explained in Chapter 2, this culminated in the 2004 Mexico Statement on Health Research, which argued that evidence derived from scientific investigation should guide health policy-making decisions, with the most effective and cost-effective interventions being adopted. This is relevant to the discussion insofar as the evidence base for behavioral HIV prevention has always been very slight—as will be shown—which therefore places a particular burden on any attempt to develop evidence-based policies in this arena.

The focus of the chapter is specifically on behavioral interventions for HIV prevention. As the name suggests, these focus on molding individuals' sexual behavior patterns so as to reduce their risk of either acquiring or transmitting HIV. Behavioral interventions are invariably concerned, one way or another, with one or more of three specific behaviors: abstinence, faithfulness, and condom use. They are also usually promoted through what are known as IEC (Information, Education, and Communication) strategies, which can take any number of forms, from mass, government-sponsored public awareness campaigns to one-to-one peer education. A number of clinic-based approaches to HIV prevention are also currently practiced, including STD management, male circumcision, counseling and testing for HIV, the provision of antiretroviral therapy (ART) to prevent mother-to-child transmission, and post-exposure antiretroviral prophylaxis. Of these, STD management as a strategy for HIV prevention has been in use in many countries since the mid-1990s, with the other approaches emerging as significant alternatives much more recently. Unlike behavioral interventions, therefore, clinic-based HIV prevention has not played a major role in AIDS control throughout the course of the whole epidemic.

After an introduction to the three central behavioral concepts—abstinence, faithfulness, and condom use—the chapter is structured into three main sections. Each of these describes a discrete epidemiological era, each of which was also characterized by a particular focus on one or other strategy for behavioral HIV prevention. These eras, and their respective HIV prevention strategies were as follows:

1. 1986 to 1992, which saw rising HIV incidence and prevalence, and a homegrown Ugandan strategy for HIV risk reduction focusing on faithfulness;
2. 1992 to 2002, a period of falling HIV incidence and prevalence alongside an increasingly open policy toward condom promotion; and
3. 2002 to 2005, in which HIV incidence and prevalence remained at a steady, relatively low level, and in which a huge influx of funds for AIDS control coincided with a rancorous international debate about the relative effectiveness of abstinence and condom use in Uganda.

Three Key Concepts: Abstinence, Faithfulness, and Condom Use

Before introducing the chapter's empirical material, it would be helpful first to briefly explore the three concepts that will be at the core of the discussion. Experience with other STDs made it clear right from the start of the AIDS epidemic that only three viable individual-level behaviors could effectively reduce the risk of sexual HIV transmission.[1] These are (i) abstinence, (ii) faithfulness to one's partner or partners,[2] and (iii) condom use. Although these are widely used terms in HIV prevention, they are often discussed without clear definitions. Clarity is essential with such topics, as illustrated by one of my respondents, a long-term expatriate social scientist living in Kampala. Describing an investigation into abstinence in rural Masaka during the early 1990s, he told me that, "we asked people [what they understood by the term abstinence], and 80 percent of what they said included sexual activity: withdrawal, condom use, one partner at a time, and sex with people who you didn't know." It is clearly a prerequisite for any discussion about a potentially controversial term to agree upon what that term actually means.

Broadly speaking, the word "abstinence" implies self-denial or restraint, and in its purest form suggests that an individual completely refrains from participating in a given activity—for example, drinking alcohol or having sex. Within the framework of HIV prevention, abstinence has usually been targeted at teenagers, by encouraging the delay of sexual debut until such time as a long-term, monogamous partner—usually a spouse—may be found. This is termed primary abstinence. Different circumstances can lead to secondary abstinence, which occurs when an individual of any age has been sexually active and then stops.

While secondary abstinence is not a major target of HIV prevention interventions—the distinction is rarely made at all—there are a number of arguments for promoting primary abstinence. These are based on moral, biological, and behavioral premises. The moral concerns, often advocated by religious groups, focus on the importance of proscribing any sort of sexual activity between people who are not married—which includes most adolescents. The main biological justification for abstinence is based on the fact that an adolescent girl's cervix matures as she grows, rendering her less susceptible to HIV infection. Behaviorally, abstinence may be beneficial because older teenagers starting to have sex may be more likely to use condoms than younger teenagers doing the same, which can further reduce the risk of infection.

As with abstinence, shades of grey also exist in the definition of the second key concept: faithfulness. Faithfulness can refer equally to one lifetime partner or to those involved in polygamous marital relationships. A less rigorous interpretation can include those who engage in serial monogamy, whereby the number of partners over an extended period may be reduced. Less rigorous still is the idea of concurrent partner reduction, whereby a person may try to have fewer coexisting sexual partners than he/she previously did. As explained over the following pages, Uganda developed a beautifully simple HIV prevention concept early in the epidemic that sought to embrace all these variations.

The third of the key topics to be discussed in this chapter—the condom—is often referred to as a modern preventive technology, but it has in fact been around for centuries. The first trial of condom efficacy was undertaken by the Italian anatomist Gabriello Fallopio in 1564, who found that none of the 1,100 men who used a linen sheath in his experiment contracted syphilis (Youssef, 1993). Since then, the condom in its various guises has been used as a means of preventing both pregnancy and the transmission of disease. The discussion here will focus exclusively on the male condom—the female condom has never featured strongly in Uganda.[3]

There is an important point about condoms that should be borne in mind throughout this chapter. The proportion of a population that reports having used a condom—either ever, or with their previous casual partner—is frequently used as a marker in the evaluation of HIV prevention interventions. An increase in these variables is usually taken to represent success for HIV prevention programs, as it suggests that people have recognized they are at risk, and have decided to take action to reduce that risk. However, while using a condom, as opposed to not using one, may be seen as protective, theories of individual risk management suggest that if a safety measure is put in place—condom use, for example, or seat belts in cars—people may compensate by taking more risk in another related area: for example, sex with a one-night stand, or driving faster (Richens et al., 2000; Adams and Hillman, 2001; Cassell et al., 2006). In this sense, condom use actually points in both directions as a marker for risk. It suggests that people recognize the danger of unprotected sex and want to reduce that danger, but they may simultaneously compensate for that risk reduction by having sex with someone they would otherwise have avoided. This makes program evaluation extremely complex. How does one rate an HIV prevention intervention that led to an increase in condom use *and* to an increase in the number of sexual partners that people were having?

This analytical problem can be further exacerbated by another related issue inherent in all survey-based sexual behavior research: the fact that people tend to misreport what they actually do in the bedroom (Dare and Cleland, 1994; Konings et al., 1995; Buvé et al., 2001; van den Borne, 2005). A respondent might have very good reasons for telling an interviewer that they used a condom when they did not, for example, or for saying they did not use a condom when they did. There are ways to improve data validity and reliability for this sort of research (Goodrich et al., 1998), but the point to bear in mind is that sexual behavior data should never be taken at face value. This is a critical issue in the context of evidence-based policy making for HIV prevention.

(i) 1986 to 1992—A Homegrown Approach to HIV Prevention

An open AIDS policy

As noted in Chapter 3, the fledgling Ugandan national ACP was established in 1986, as a department of the Ministry of Health. It was the first ACP in Africa and was manned by a dozen professional staff, who in turn were assisted by five technical specialists from WHO. The ACP's mandate included four main areas:

1. Health education (in the form of IEC);
2. Surveillance of the epidemic;
3. Ensuring a safe blood transfusion supply; and
4. Improving patient care.

A significant amount of money was required to set up such an ambitious national program from scratch—especially given the crumbling state of the health infrastructure after so many long years of war—so a donors' conference was held in June 1987, at which a sum of $7.4 million was pledged to run the first year of operations (ACP, 1989a:5). As a senior official in the Ministry of Health nostalgically quipped, "the donors were very soft then, very user-friendly," so the government was able to receive strong financial support. Reliable estimates of national HIV prevalence rates were not yet available, but the huge scale of the epidemic was illustrated by the fact that 25 percent of antenatal mothers attending the national referral hospital at Mulago, Kampala, tested HIV-positive in 1988 (ACP, 1991:14).

The backdrop to all the ACP's work was one core principle: that Uganda would pursue an open policy toward AIDS. In the words of the Ministry official quoted above, "the key person was the President, and he guaranteed that the government's position would be open, frank, positive, and proactive in dealing with it." This openness included the demand that elected officials from national level all the way down to village level brought AIDS into their discussions at every public meeting. Uganda's AIDS policy was quickly recognized and praised on the international stage: one author wrote as early as 1989 that "Uganda is probably the African country most open about the scale of its AIDS problem" (Anderson, 1989:8).

But apart from revealing the scale of the problem and talking about it, what did it actually mean to be "open"? And why would the President opt for such a policy? A Ugandan social scientist saw Museveni's response primarily as pragmatism in the face of an overwhelming emergency: "I think the openness was because maybe the government wanted to get assistance. Maybe—how shall I put it?—being open is not being open for the sake of being open. It is being open because you can't manage the problem, and you want other people to come and help . . . It has helped a lot because foreign agencies have come in to do research and bring in money for interventions and care and all that. It has done something, but I think the openness was for other reasons than being open."

However, not every aspect of Uganda's AIDS policy was open at that stage. As an outspoken advocate for urgent action in the face of the epidemic, Wilson Carswell—the Scottish surgeon who led the first AIDS research in the country, as described in Chapter 3—was declared persona non grata and deported in April 1987. Also, two of his servants were murdered at his Kampala house in March 1987, by people he claims to have been from Military Intelligence. Given the purported open policy, I asked him why he thought this had happened. "I was saying that a lot of them would die," he replied, "and that was seen as negative. To say that a lot of people would die was [seen as] the same as saying that I wish a lot would die." Regardless of who may or may not have been responsible, it would appear that there was a dark side to the politics of AIDS in Uganda during that period, and that complete openness was not necessarily always welcome.

Education—a vaccine for AIDS

At that early stage in the epidemic, a positive test for HIV spelled doom for an infected person. Treatment of AIDS-related opportunistic infections was of limited effectiveness, and prevention of infection remained the only long-term means of combating the virus. Behavior change thus became the main pillar of control efforts. To this end, Peter Piot—then a scientist at the Institute of Tropical Medicine in Antwerp, but subsequently Executive Director of UNAIDS—wrote in 1987 that "the main thrust of control [worldwide] must be education of all sexually active young men and women. Education about HIV must begin now" (Piot et al., 1987:203).

The question in Uganda was exactly what form that education would take. According to an expatriate advisor, "the policy at that stage was simply to inform. During the time when I was with the ACP, the policy was information: 'Tell people, and then the instinct for self preservation will help them avoid it.'" Responsibility for behavior change was thereby passed to individuals, with no recognition of the wider structural issues—such as gender inequality and poverty—that later research suggested can affect people's ability to engage in safer sexual behavior. This point is clearly made by the contents of an editorial message in an ACP surveillance report from 1989, which addressed health care workers and administrators: "The information contained in this report gives you a clear picture of the AIDS situation in Uganda. It is not meant to frighten you. Knowledge is power. Now that you have information about AIDS, you are empowered to consciously decide to abstain from irresponsible and unhealthy sexual relationships, and similarly educate others . . . The decision to save your life is entirely yours. We wish you good reading" (ACP, 1989b:1).

AIDS information was disseminated to the general population through many channels, with full use made of the existing infrastructure. Thus, Resistance Councils,[4] churches and mosques, and, to some extent, schools were engaged. The mass media also contributed significantly, with Radio Uganda employing an AIDS team that was responsible for transmitting messages in six languages before and after every news bulletin, punctuated with the dramatic use of traditional drums. Theatre groups toured their local areas performing plays about AIDS; and in 1989, a Ugandan musician who himself had AIDS—Philly Lutaaya—became the first public figure in the country to openly declare his status. "There was a lot of singing about AIDS in those days," an English former volunteer worker in Masaka told me, "and it was very emotional. Philly Lutaaya's song was, 'Today it's me, tomorrow it's someone else.' It had a big impact." Meanwhile, UNICEF was engaged with the Ministry of Health in the production of leaflets, posters, and other awareness-raising items: by 1989, close to seven million pamphlets and four tons of badges and stickers had been distributed (ACP, 1989a:8). Collectively, therefore, a huge effort was made nationwide during the late 1980s to educate the Ugandan population about AIDS.

But what were the messages that were actually being put out? Much of the initial focus was on providing basic facts regarding how HIV is transmitted and how it is not transmitted. This proved to be an ongoing task that would last for many years: people continued for a long time to be concerned about transmission through everyday, nonsexual contact, and about the possible danger of infection via mosquitoes (ACP, 1989a:4; ACP, 1992:2). Such concerns had to be dispelled, not least because people living with AIDS could otherwise be isolated and stigmatized, and might fail to receive the care and support that they needed at home (Konde Lule et al., 1989).

With the basic facts about transmission widely publicized, it was important also to develop messages that would help people to protect themselves from infection. Research suggested heterosexual transmission of HIV was responsible for 90 percent of infections in Uganda (ACP, 1989a:4), information that subsequently facilitated the identification of the three viable behaviors that can protect an individual from this mode of HIV transmission. As described above, these were: (i) avoid sexual contact altogether or abstain; (ii) stick to (one) mutually faithful, HIV-negative partner(s); or (iii) use a condom if engaging in sex outside the context of (ii).

The task of policy makers was then to select the relative emphasis of these three behaviors. Decisions were made fast, with the country's early HIV prevention strategy explained in 1987 by Dr. Sam Okware, then head of the ACP: "The key thing is to love carefully and have zero grazing . . . Condoms are a problem because of our cultural beliefs and traditions. My people do not use condoms and do not want to use condoms so we do not promote them as a method of stopping AIDS. In Uganda condoms are associated with prostitution so most people would not use them. If we ordered people to wear condoms they would not accept it, and we don't want to give the population the false hope that the condom is 100 percent safe . . . because it isn't. Why should we encourage people to get false confidence?" (*Sydney Morning Herald*, 1987).

Thus the government's position was clear from the start: condoms were out, and zero-grazing—a familiar concept to everyone in Uganda's predominantly agrarian society—was in. People were advised to avoid the virus by grazing, sexually speaking, exclusively within their own paddock, and to curtail any free-range activities. Such a concept is in many ways the Holy Grail of health promotion, since it takes a widely understood idea and puts an unusual, humorous slant on it, thereby rendering it inherently memorable. A British journalist in Kampala during the late 1980s agreed with this point, telling me that "the concept of zero-grazing was talked about, laughed about. Baganda people liked that double talk." But an expatriate social scientist was not so convinced: "'Stick to one partner' also meant to many people 'stuck with one partner,'" he told me. "Nobody was talking about having an interesting and fulfilling sexual life, with variety and spice. It was all about *don't!*"

The government's push for zero-grazing was also supplemented by the promotion of abstinence, largely by faith-based groups. The late Bishop Adrian Ddungu, formerly Bishop of Masaka Diocese, explained to me before his final illness that "at the beginning of the present government, the President stressed the idea of abstinence. He very often gave an example of an anthill which usually has holes near it and advised against putting one's hand into these holes because snakes are most likely to take shelter there. At that time, the President and the Church saw things eye to eye."

Thus the strategy had been set, but many people were nonetheless skeptical about its effectiveness. Even the ACP itself was not satisfied, berating the population in a surveillance report editorial from 1990, and saying that "much of this knowledge has been misinterpreted by society for convenience. Most have taken a faithful partner to mean having two or three partners. Those already caught up in polygamous marriages may perhaps be excused. One only hopes that they will have the sense to zero-graze within that setting only" (ACP, 1990:1). Anecdotal evidence confirms the misinterpretation of this knowledge. A former NGO worker told me that "on the message of limiting sexual partners, the joke was that this meant 'one wife in this town, one in Kampala, one at home etc'"; and an expatriate AIDS epidemiologist referred to the behavior of his survey team while working in the field: "With the guys at the end of the day, it was 'OK, where are the ladies?'"

An Assistant Commissioner at the Ministry of Health also spoke of the struggle to put the messages across: "When we started talking about abstinence, zero-grazing and so on, nobody used to take us seriously. Before the news on the radio, there was a jingle with drums, and it was always followed by a message about AIDS. But people would turn down the radio when they heard the jingle, and then turn it up when the news started. They didn't take us seriously. So we used to go to meet His Excellency and he would abuse us because there was no change in the people. But we are dealing with people who are dynamic. It takes *time*." His thoughts are supported by the conclusions of a study published in 1989, which said that "information about the AIDS epidemic is reaching the Ugandan population; however, changes in behavior are slower to follow" (Konde Lule et al., 1989:517; see also Kirumira, 1992).

Thus there was concern in many quarters about the effectiveness of the campaign. But, as will become clear over the following pages, very little useable research evidence was available at the time to guide policy makers toward more effective approaches. And in the absence of evidence, there had been no choice but to base Uganda's HIV prevention strategy on the hunch that condoms would inevitably prove unpopular, and that therefore people should strive toward zero-grazing and abstinence instead.

The role of the Catholic Church in Masaka

One of the predominant characteristics of southwestern Uganda is the high proportion of the population that is Roman Catholic: according to the Church itself, 75 percent of the people of Masaka considered themselves to be Catholics in the year 1990 (Catholic Hierarchy, 2006). With the Church's very particular stance on contraception, AIDS would provide an important barometer of its evolving strategy for dealing with issues relating to sexuality. And with Masaka Diocese as the site of the world's first community-wide AIDS epidemic, the Catholic authorities there could potentially play a significant role in defining the response for other parts of Africa and the world. I asked the two bishops who have held the seat since the start of the epidemic—Bishop Adrian Ddungu, who led the Catholic flock in Masaka from 1962 to 1998; and Bishop John Baptist Kaggwa, the present incumbent—about the principles and evidence that had guided their response to AIDS.

Bishop Kaggwa described how his predecessor had reacted to AIDS when the epidemic first emerged. "There was no medicine, so he started waging his campaign by opening people's eyes. All the sermons in the churches were about awareness, about the causes of AIDS, about transmission. So he sensitized everyone, also using youth groups, through plays and songs."

I asked the Bishop what the message had been. "The message was that the disease has come, there is no medicine, and that contracting it leads to death. But you can avoid it, because transmission is through sex, so you must love carefully and consciously. Which means faithfulness to your partner, or to wait for mature times. Abstinence was very strongly encouraged. And those who paid heed were saved. Of course there are other ways of reducing AIDS, such as condoms. But we strongly advise our people to use the method of abstinence. It is more effective, and more dignified: it creates character. We are not looking only at AIDS control. We're looking at the person, at the changing of society. So once he [Bishop Ddungu] knew the transmission mechanisms of AIDS, he realized the only possible thing to do was to abstain, unless you're married. It was very hard for him to see his people dying like rats."

What about condoms? Could they ever have a role to play? "I was at a meeting," he explained, "and the medical doctors who were talking about AIDS made an experiment. They filled a condom with pepper, and then asked if people could feel the pepper through the condom. I didn't do it myself, but some of the others did. And they could feel the pepper. So then we concluded that if pepper can seep through, what about the virus, which is much smaller? So then we concluded that the condoms we have now are not protective against HIV. They may be good for family planning, but not for anti-virus. The Vatican uses this evidence to show that the condom is not a good method of prevention. Ninety seven percent of all condoms, the virus can go through. And you don't know which is the lucky three percent. So how can we promote something that we know is not effective?"

I met Bishop Ddungu himself a few weeks later, and asked for his view on the condom as a means for preventing HIV. He also turned to the evidence he had used to substantiate his position, which proved to be remarkably similar in essence to that used by Kaggwa. "The scientific research made available and strengthened by our medical services has been very helpful," he replied. "It is, however, very unfortunate that outside our own circles the use of condoms has been overstressed. A team of a doctor from South Africa and a Benedictine priest from USA came here and gave us some lectures on HIV/AIDS. They showed us slides, amongst other things, and made it clear that the sperm and gonorrhea mucus, which is thicker than that of HIV/AIDS, can go through the condom. Therefore it is not clear how a condom can be impermeable to HIV/AIDS substance, which is smaller than the above. The use of condoms has been unnecessarily stressed."

The message from both bishops, therefore, was that condoms should be avoided first and foremost on moral grounds, but also on the basis of what they deemed to be convincing experimental evidence.

Since Bishop Ddungu had been present at the very start of the African AIDS epidemic, I also asked him whether there was ever any exchange of ideas between himself and the Vatican about the approach that should be taken toward HIV prevention. In other words, who had influence over whom?

"We give a talk each time we go [to Rome],"[5] he replied, "to give them an idea of what we are doing. They give us instructions and advice. But we did mention about AIDS in the Congregation for the Propagation of the Faith. Also there's a Council that has something to do with health—we gave them something about the situation, how we were dealing with this disease. But I don't remember them looking for advice from me, on policy. Within the Church there was not much discussion about the approach to be taken against AIDS. You have the Commandments: Thou shalt not kill, and Thou shalt not commit adultery. Internally, we never had a disagreement. From the start, it was clear that the Church would stand against condoms. We didn't need to ask them about it; it was taken for granted."

Thus there was neither disagreement nor debate within the Catholic hierarchy about how people should avoid HIV, a point that is further emphasized by the following official message from the Catholic Bishops of Uganda, published in September 1989. "A Christian who lives and acts with faith under the guidance of the Spirit will practice the virtues of chastity, conjugal fidelity and self-mastery and control, because he knows that these are the only ways that are in conformity with human dignity capable of leading him to a more complete and balanced development and to a greater happiness . . . Apart from the fact that condoms which are being promoted by some agencies only reduce the risk and are not a guarantee against the acquiring of AIDS, their use as a means to avoid the disease is unacceptable from the moral point of view. Indeed, having recourse to this method ignores the real cause that occupies us, namely the permissiveness that corrodes the moral fiber of the people" (Catholic Bishops of Uganda, 1989:10–11).

Both bishops—as well as the wider Catholic community in Uganda— therefore held clear views about the appropriate means of protecting oneself against HIV, with the "moral" position taking precedence, and with condoms considered to be absolutely unacceptable. It is striking that the government and the Catholic lines were remarkably similar at that stage: anti-condom, pro-fidelity, and pro-abstinence.

A change in strategy—quiet condom promotion begins

The official line changed in early 1991, however, with "a reluctant pledge by President Yoweri Museveni to advocate condom use" (Tebere, 1991:3). The President's change of heart had been prompted in the face of alarming new figures released by the ACP that showed a continued increase in HIV infection rates: HIV prevalence among antenatal mothers attending the national referral hospital in Kampala had risen from 25 percent in 1988 to 39 percent in 1990, and an estimated 1.5 million Ugandans were now believed to be infected (ACP, 1991). Museveni was clearly rattled by the data. In June 1991, he gave the keynote address at the Seventh International Conference on AIDS, held in Florence, during which he grimly announced that Africa faced an "apocalypse" (Barnett and Blaikie, 1992:152).

In spite of the worrying surveillance data, the policy change to advocate condom use was nonetheless difficult and controversial. As an Entebbe-based scientist explained, "there was a conflict between the condom pro-moters—who were basically WHO and the expatriate community—and the Catholic Church. Museveni was basically against condoms, but he recognized their value in the short term, while people became less profligate."

Vincent Ssempijja, currently Chairman of Masaka district, was involved in some of the discussions, and he spoke of how the conflict was resolved by necessity. "We met the bishops many times," he told me, "and I remember they were very bitter about it. But at the end of the day, the government agreed that we lead sinners, we lead the faithful ones, we lead those very good people, we lead thieves, and we know that there are also accidents, that there are people who can catch AIDS from accidents. So we know we have all of them. And a sinner today may not be a sinner tomorrow; and this sinner may be an engineer and we need him to do other things. So condom promotion became part of the policy." This new policy dictated that abstinence and zero-grazing would continue to predominate, but "quiet" condom promotion—via social marketing strategies (as explained below) though not through the official media—would be permitted.

Meanwhile, another important policy change emerged. The ever-expanding nature of the epidemic convinced Museveni and his advisors that the health sector could not cope alone, and thus Uganda became the first African country to establish a multisectoral approach to AIDS control. The Uganda AIDS Commission (UAC) was set up by a statute of Parliament in 1992, "to oversee, plan and co-ordinate AIDS prevention and control activities throughout Uganda, and in particular to formulate policy and establish programmatic priorities" (UAC, 1992:5). The Uganda AIDS Commission was placed under the direct supervision of the President, and it was explicitly charged with seeking to tackle the social and economic causes and consequences of the AIDS epidemic.

The role of research in developing Uganda's early HIV prevention policy

One of the conclusions of the Fifth International AIDS Conference held in Montreal in 1989 was that "much African social research, whether psychological or anthropological, tends to be descriptive, and research on factors that motivate behavioural risk reduction is required. Evaluation of mass campaigns and high risk group interventions alike must complement self-reports with other data, especially on STDs" (Wilson, 1989:198). This important point was apparently overlooked by the research community, as it was repeated again the following year, after the Sixth International AIDS Conference, in San Francisco: "It is hoped that post-San Francisco activities . . . will emphasize interventions, action research and research linked to interventions" (Wilson and Lavelle, 1990:375).

Most of the scientific work being conducted at that stage consisted of "numbing sero-epidemiologies of urban, convenience samples" (ibid.:371), which meant that the epidemic in rural areas—where most African people live and where the burden of disease has always been predominantly felt—was very poorly understood. Nonetheless, such epidemiological studies conducted early on by Carswell and colleagues had established that AIDS in Uganda was predominantly heterosexually transmitted (Sewankambo et al., 1987), a crucial first step in identifying possible prevention interventions. The heterosexual transmissibility of HIV was not as self-evident as it may appear today: a senior UNAIDS executive told me how one of the reviewers for a paper he submitted to the *Lancet* in the late 1980s wrote that "it's a well known fact that AIDS cannot be transmitted from women to men."

Aside from the recognition of heterosexual HIV transmission, and the associated high risk groups such as sex workers, barmaids, and truck drivers (Carswell, 1987), there was effectively no evidence from anywhere in Africa to substantiate programmatic or policy decisions with regards to which particular HIV prevention strategies—abstinence, zero-grazing, or condom use—should be stressed. The epidemic was, after all, still very young, and there had been no time to conduct studies to evaluate different intervention approaches. Without substantive evaluations, decisions were inevitably therefore based on a hunch, on common sense, or on moral ideology. Such an approach was, in fact, common practice at that time: several years would pass before the concept of evidence-based policy making emerged.

The need for a scientific basis from which to respond to AIDS had nonetheless been recognized in Uganda, with an invitation to the British Medical Research Council (MRC) to establish a long-term AIDS research program in a rural part of the country. The MRC Programme on AIDS subsequently opened its doors in Entebbe on 15 August 1988, with two epidemiologists—one Ugandan and one Dutch—occupying a small office at the Uganda Virus Research Institute (UVRI). The MRC's mandate included "operational epidemiological studies . . . with emphasis on search for cofactors responsible for transmission. Appropriate social studies will be undertaken as well to look for social behaviour which encourage transmission" (ACP, 1991:21–22). Historically, UVRI had focused on arbovirus research, and although the facilities were in a state of some neglect, the Institute had managed to avoid the widespread looting that had taken place throughout much of the country during the war. In the words of a scientist who once worked there, "any soldier knew that there were dangerous pathogens lurking in the freezers." With its history of viral research and relatively intact facilities, "the Virus"—as it is locally known—was therefore a straightforward choice at which to establish the new Programme's headquarters.

The two epidemiologists spent their first year identifying possible sites in Masaka district for setting up a cohort in order to conduct a longitudinal study[6] of the epidemic's dynamics. The hope was that, as the epidemic evolved, the cohort would provide a detailed understanding of changing HIV infection and associated mortality rates, as well as of sexual behavior patterns. After extensive groundwork, a rural sub-county in the north of rural Masaka district called Kyamulibwa was finally identified, about

140 kilometers from the MRC's Entebbe offices. Over 4,000 people in the sub-county were interviewed and bled in the first annual sero-survey in 1989, which demonstrated an overall HIV prevalence rate of 8.2 percent (Kamali et al., 2000). The data showed strong variations by age and sex, with the highest prevalence being found in women aged 20–24 (21 percent HIV positive), and in men aged 25–34 (18 percent).

The situation was, however, considerably worse in neighboring Rakai district. A U.S.-funded research group that had been established there in 1988—the Rakai Project—reported overall adult HIV prevalence rates in its cohort for 1990 of 35 percent in main road trading centers, 23 percent in trading villages situated on secondary roads, and 12 percent in rural agrarian villages (Sewankambo et al., 1994). Not only was there great variability in prevalence within a relatively small geographical area, therefore, but these population-based surveys also confirmed the disastrous scale of the epidemic in this corner of Uganda.

I asked an expatriate scientist who had been involved at the time how study topics had been decided upon by the MRC and the Rakai Project. "Lots of cross-fertilization of ideas took place across the dinner table in Entebbe," she told me, adding that personal relationships between staff from the two organizations stimulated the development of research topics much more than any discussion with people in the study communities— even if relations between researchers and the study communities were generally cordial. None of the work at that stage concerned the evaluation of HIV prevention interventions.[7]

"We were very insular," she continued, "and focused on publication to prove that the research was productive. Our interaction with local government was more to do with the acceptability of the research than with the issue itself." I asked if any of her research findings had had any sort of impact on policy or programs in Uganda. "It did have an impact on [her organization's funder], since they were very pleased that people were actually talking about our work in meetings. But did it have an effect on anything that was actually being done on the ground? No."

Another former researcher concurred: "The impact of research on policy? Pretty well removed. But it did create its own little industry and a visible presence, by giving donors and embassies something to support. People said, 'the *bazungu*[8] really do think this is important. It's not just a flash in the pan.'" This visible presence was apparently very important for people living in the study communities, as well as for many of the Ugandan researchers involved. Community leaders wanted some sort of infrastructure to be provided, specifically curative services; and one senior Ugandan researcher in particular was constantly asking his expatriate colleagues: "What are you going to do for Uganda today?" His particular concern was with trying to have Ugandan staff trained up to a high level, specifically through Masters courses abroad.

Although President Museveni himself had played a part in inviting the two research programs into the country, one respondent told me that this was not so much because of the important research being conducted, but rather because the organizations' presence gave him credibility. Uganda—and by proxy, Museveni himself—was being rewarded for its openness about AIDS. Museveni reportedly had other interests in addition to the science in mind, even though, as my respondent said, "his recognition of the research projects being done there was fulsome."

Formal research may have had limited impact on AIDS policy or on programmatic design, therefore, perhaps partly because this did not always seem to be a top priority either for the researchers themselves, or for the President—the country's top policy maker. Likewise, the monitoring and evaluation conducted by many non-research-based implementing agencies was also incomplete. One respondent who had worked on a project during the late 1980s complained to me that "they [the donors] don't want to know your dirty laundry; they want to know about successes, lessons learned." As a result, she said, "we couldn't really prove we'd made an impact, other than being part of a network." Another respondent working with TASO[9]—the country's largest non-governmental AIDS service provider and a major recipient of foreign aid—said that their evaluation process was "more about project management than about what works. It was more monitoring and audit: how many and how often." Justifying funds received from donors thus became an important activity in its own right. As she explained, "by 1989, [AIDS in Uganda] had become a sort of feeding ground for the international agencies—and money distorts things."

Overall, the research conducted during the late 1980s—whether formal scientific investigations or programmatic monitoring and evaluation—appeared not to have been especially useful. I therefore asked several respondents whether they had ever been aware of their own research being taken into account during any decision making process. The responses suggested something of a grey area.

One senior Ugandan scientist told me about the "concerted efforts we made to interface with policy makers. I don't know if we influenced them, but they asked good questions," she said, adding that "they too were very worried about what was going on." She also said that every article that was submitted for publication had to pass through the Ministry of Health for approval, "and I suppose they read them before approving them." Furthermore, she recalled organizing a small scientific meeting in

Kampala, "and the press picked it up, so things appeared in the papers, and these were read. The issue of circumcision[10] came up in the papers, and suddenly everyone was saying 'the Moslems are safe from AIDS!' But this was all informal, nothing that I could say, yes, this scientific result led to this policy."

A similar line of argument was taken by a former Makerere University–based social scientist, and one of the very first people to become engaged in investigating Uganda's AIDS epidemic. Although her work in the 1980s may not have had a direct effect on policy or practice, she told me that it "opened up other questions for exploration: issues about partner relationships and gender that nobody else was asking about then; the way women with AIDS are treated in the home, as compared to the way that men with AIDS are treated. Also economic aspects—and I think this may be one of the reasons that [South African President] Mbeki is so strongly talking about poverty and AIDS. We brought out this issue first in 1989. At that time, nobody was asking these questions. So this was being picked up by students, and shaping their minds—the minds of future policy makers—and they went out afterwards much more sensitive to the issues." She conceded that her thoughts on this are speculative, and that finding any certain evidence of any work having a definitive impact on policy is difficult. She did feel, however, that the effect was cumulative: "There wasn't any one study that made an impact, but our data laid a foundation in 1989, and by 1995 it was being taken up by WHO."

With the exceptions of the initial epidemiological studies that established that HIV in Uganda was heterosexually transmitted, and the surveillance data presented by the ACP to President Museveni in 1991—that pushed him reluctantly toward the quiet condom promotion policy—we can conclude that research played a very minor role in defining AIDS control policy and practice during the period 1986 to 1992. This applies both to the official government response as well as to influential authorities within the Roman Catholic Church. One reason was of course the fact that past a certain point, much of the research being conducted—the "numbing sero-epidemiologies" conducted in easily accessed urban areas—was of limited value for policy makers or program designers. And while this sort of research was being conducted, HIV prevalence continued to climb at a terrible rate.

As it happens, however, the period around 1991 marked the zenith of the AIDS epidemic in Masaka and, broadly speaking, in Uganda as a whole. Data from the MRC show falling HIV incidence from this point, which means that people had collectively started to change their sexual behavior, and that the tide had turned.

(ii) 1992 to 2002—The Rise of the Condom

Condoms, controversy, and the growth of Uganda's AIDS industry

The advent of Uganda's quiet condom promotion policy in 1991 marked a substantial change in the country's overall strategy to control HIV. Condoms were then still only available via family planning clinics and some pharmacies. Fewer than 10 million had been brought into the country since the establishment of the ACP five years earlier, in 1986 (*New York Times*, 1991); and a survey conducted in Rakai district in 1988–89 found that no more than 2 percent of 1,292 respondents reported ever having used a condom (Rakai Project, 1991:3). This low figure can be attributed to both very limited supply and very limited demand.

But as part of a $12 million HIV prevention grant to Uganda from USAID—for many years the single biggest provider of condoms to developing countries—came funds intended to find out specifically how best to package and sell condoms in the country Perlez (*New York Times*, 1991). Social marketing principles[11] similar to those that had already been successfully adopted for condom promotion by USAID in neighboring Zaire were to be taken as a starting point, the overall idea being first to create a demand for condoms, and then to meet that demand. Both the private and the public sectors were to be involved.

As explained above, however, there was a great deal of opposition to the condom in Uganda at the time, with many people associating their use with promiscuity and prostitution. Furthermore, one of my respondents—a man from rural Masaka—added that, "at first, people didn't want to use condoms. They had this belief that the *bazungu*[12] are very clever. They want Africans to die, so they put the virus inside the condom. And if you use it, you will get the virus, because of that oil they put on the condom. They ask, have you ever heard of these Europeans who die from AIDS? They don't die of AIDS. We Africans are the only people who die of AIDS." A primary task of the social marketers, therefore, was to address such perceptions.

The first brand—Protector condoms—appeared in 1991, and an advertisement in a national newspaper from that year shows the care that was being taken in promoting the product. Alongside the words "Be wise— always wear Protector condoms" is a picture of a smiling, thoroughly respectable-looking couple (*Weekly Topic*, 1991:10). Protector condoms were being sold on the basis of their being sensible, safe products—a line also adopted in 1997 by Life Guard condoms,[13] which were advertised on the basis that "condoms are the only sure way of reducing the risks of unplanned pregnancy and sexually transmitted diseases, including HIV/AIDS"

(Life Guard, 1997). Given that abstaining from sex altogether is in fact the only sure way to reduce these risks, this was a little disingenuous, but the determination of the social marketers to promote their product is undeniable.

It was not until the late 1990s that Uganda's condom social marketers felt confident enough to promote their product as fun and sexy. One such advertisement for Life Guard condoms appeared in 1999, featuring a well-muscled man in shorts carrying a woman draped scantily in a cloth, with a waterfall as a backdrop. I recall that a billboard with this advertisement was placed at a strategically busy corner in Nyendo—a low-income township outside Masaka—but there was uproar when it emerged that the land on which it had been placed belonged to the Catholic Church. The billboard was quickly taken down.

At the local level, the potential of condom social marketing was illustrated by work conducted during the MRC's Masaka Intervention Trial (MIT), an evaluation of two different HIV prevention strategies.[14] An initial assessment of the study areas throughout rural Masaka conducted in 1994, found significant misconceptions about and opposition to condoms from the general community, and also that small retailers feared ridicule and a loss of clientele if they stocked condoms. But after five years of intensive community-based condom promotion (1995–1999 inclusive), during which donor-subsidized condoms that permitted a 100 percent profit margin for retailers were provided, 1.5 million condoms had been sold to a population of approximately 96,000 adults. Misconceptions and opposition had also significantly decreased (Basajja et al., 2000). The conclusion was that the local-level social marketing of condoms through commercial channels had effectively improved their acceptability, availability, and accessibility to this rural community. The planned approach to social change had largely succeeded, and had done so relatively fast.

On a much larger scale, major new actors such as the World Bank were also entering the fray for the first time. Following on from its groundbreaking 1993 World Development Report (World Bank, 1993)—which, in a departure from previously held positions, highlighted the role of health in economic development—the Bank financed a six-year STI[15] Project in Uganda, to the tune of $73 million (World Bank, 2003). The STI Project ran from 1994, and included a significant condom promotion component in addition to its other activities related to sexually transmitted infections and HIV. World Bank–funded condoms were distributed for free, via the public sector.

Uganda's condom promotion program grew significantly during these years. Distribution increased from the woefully low levels indicated above during the late 1980s to 4 million socially marketed condoms in 1994, and up to 16 million in 1997 (DKT International, 2006; see also Thornton, 2008:144), with a similar number distributed for free through the public sector.

This increased programmatic activity was not, however, reflected in the policy arena. As mentioned above, the Uganda AIDS Commission had been placed in charge of AIDS policy development for the country in 1992, but a draft set of policy proposals written in April 1995 conceded that "there are so far no articulated national policies on AIDS control" (UAC, 1995:11). This policy proposal document—part of a consultation exercise to develop a comprehensive set of national policies—included discussion of 34 policy issues, of which condoms were first on the list. Quiet condom promotion remained as a de facto, unwritten policy, and the policy proposal was intended to formalize this by "promot[ing] responsible use of condoms based on appropriate education and training" (ibid.:13). However, this policy proposal document never went further than circulation and discussion. One Member of Parliament complained in July 1997 that although operational guidelines were in place for HIV testing, surveillance, and patient care, "a comprehensive set of national policies is yet to be generated" (Musumba, 1997:7).

In October 1997, the unwritten policy of quiet condom promotion was scrapped by the Minister of Health, Crispus Kiyonga, who explained that the policy had "been overtaken by events" (*New Vision*, 1997a). Referring to declining rates of HIV infection in the country (as detailed below), he said that "the fall of HIV rates is largely due to condom use. There is no question that [the condom] helps." National ACP manager Dr. Elizabeth Madraa added that the government had seen "the demand by the people and had let the people decide . . . We see that those who used to be very strongly against the condom are now saying let it be used by married people, by people infected with HIV, by people who cannot abstain" (ibid.). The change in policy was not formal or written, but the new position was clear nonetheless: condom promotion could now be conducted openly, including through government media.

I asked Masaka's Bishop Ddungu why he thought the policy had been changed. "It was for political reasons," he told me. "The support we receive from outside comes with strings attached. Either you accept the condoms or we stop the aid." His strong doubts about the new policy were, not surprisingly, shared by the head of the Roman Catholic Church in Uganda, Emmanuel Cardinal Wamala, who explained to his congregation how, "I at one time approached condom dealers and inquired whether they would allow giving their children bicycles without brakes to ride since they would be carrying bandages with them. This is exactly what [condom promoters] are trying to do" (*New Vision*, 1997b). Yet this anti-condom view was not adopted by all Catholics. Dr. Speciosa Kazibwe, the Roman Catholic Vice President of Uganda, was quoted as saying that "the Cardinal [Wamala] does not allow talk on condoms, but I have to tell the people about them because [otherwise] the Cardinal would not have people to preach to" (*New Vision*, 2000a).

Emotions continued to run high on the matter, with proponents on both sides fiercely defending their ideological positions, invariably in the absence of any evidence to support any given position: this was a moral, not a scientific debate. The facts on the ground superseded the discussion, however. According to Dr. Peter Nsubuga, manager of the World Bank's STI Project, "demand [for condoms] is going through the roof, but our ability to meet this demand is not there" (*New Vision*, 2000b). The ever-increasing focus on condoms—at the expense of abstinence and zero-grazing—was such that Pastor Martin Sempa, an evangelical Christian leader, bitterly observed how, "in Kampala, the original billboards advocating for abstinence have either collapsed or rusted and a new breed of condom-promoting billboards have replaced them. The whole anti-HIV/AIDS campaign has been taken over by the commercial interest of promoting condoms" (*New Vision*, 2002a). Official figures show that around 170 million free condoms were distributed in the country between 1997 and 2002 inclusive, with an additional 117 million sold through social marketing groups (ACP, 2003:15). This translates to an average annual availability of 48 million condoms during those six years—a lot of condoms, but perhaps not so many when counted against the nation's population, in 2002, of 24 million people (Uganda Bureau of Statistics, 2002b). With approximately 50 percent of Ugandans, or 12 million people, being potentially sexually active,[16] this works out at an average of eight condoms per couple per year. As a senior official in the Ministry of Health told me, "a peasant with two or three wives may have several rounds [of sex] in one night." These eight condoms may not therefore last for very long.

Pastor Sempa was perhaps therefore exaggerating slightly, but "AIDS in Uganda" had certainly turned into a large industry. The country's AIDS control efforts were being conducted by a huge array of actors, with over 1,200 different agencies implementing all sorts of AIDS-related activities in the country in 1997 (UAC, 2002). The cost of this was substantial, with foreign donors covering most of the cost. Elizabeth Marum of the U.S. Centers for Disease Control estimated that donor support covered 70 percent of Uganda's prevention and care activities between 1989 and 1998, amounting to $180 million, or an estimated $1.80 per adult per year (Hogle et al., 2002:11).

And as the twenty-first century dawned, global interest in AIDS grew yet further, with an increasing awareness that although Uganda may have done well in reducing incidence and prevalence, many other countries in Africa—most notably in the south of the continent—were facing explosive epidemics. In April 2000, the Clinton administration described AIDS as a threat to U.S. national security and to global stability (*Independent*, 2000); and subsequently, UN Secretary General Kofi Annan convened the General Assembly in July 2001, for a Special Session on HIV/AIDS (UNGASS), the first time the General Assembly had met to discuss a health issue. One of the concrete outcomes of this meeting was the founding in January 2002, of the Global Fund to Fight AIDS, Tuberculosis and Malaria, an international organization with a remit to make large grants to countries in need of assistance in tackling these conditions. Uganda would soon become one of the Global Fund's major recipients.

The period from 1992 to 2002 can thus be described in Uganda as a time in which condom distribution and use increased relentlessly, even in the face of considerable opposition from powerful religious groups—and even though the number of condoms available per couple per year remained relatively low. Simultaneously, the emphasis on zero-grazing that had prevailed during the early years of AIDS control efforts was significantly reduced. The AIDS industry became very well established during this time, too, with tens of millions of dollars flowing in to fund programs across the country. But the enormously increased global interest in AIDS from 2000 onwards set the stage for an entirely new chapter in the history of the epidemic, a period in which the funding levels that had once seemed substantial would begin to appear rather paltry.

Epidemiological developments

The prevailing epidemiological feature of HIV in Uganda during this period of intensive condom promotion was of falling HIV prevalence; and also, in Masaka at least, falling HIV incidence. It was during the 1990s that Uganda emerged on the international stage as *the* African AIDS success story, and first efforts were made to try to establish how the country's prevention efforts were connected with what had happened epidemiologically.

Evidence began to accumulate from the mid-1990s onwards of a generalized and sustained fall in HIV prevalence in many parts of the country. The first synthesis of evidence pointing in this direction examined presentations given at the Ninth International Conference on AIDS and STD in Africa, held in Kampala in 1995. The various data sources reviewed included the general population cohorts[17] in Masaka (3.6 percent of men aged 13–24 were HIV-positive in 1990–91, falling to 1 percent in 1994–95) and Rakai (overall adult prevalence at main road trading centers fell from 38 percent in 1990 to 31 percent in 1992); as well as from antenatal clinics in Kampala (falling from 28 percent HIV-positive in 1988–89 to 16 percent in 1993). The conclusion was that "there appears to be a real decline in HIV seroprevalence in some population groups in Uganda" (Konde Lule, 1995:33).

Further supporting evidence continued to come in from all over the country over the following years, predominantly from the easiest group to monitor systematically: pregnant women. Significant declines in HIV prevalence were noted in young pregnant women in the western district of Fort Portal (Kilian et al., 1999) and several other urban centers (ACP, 1999). But the most widely representative and comprehensive data suggestive of falling HIV prevalence came from the general population cohorts in Rakai and Masaka (Wawer et al., 1997; Kamali et al., 2000).

Falling HIV prevalence is of course good news, as this means simply that fewer people are carrying the virus. But the key to controlling an HIV epidemic is in fact to reduce HIV incidence—or new infections. Prevalence is defined as the overall proportion of a population that is infected, and is a product of incidence as well as mortality and migration. Thus falling prevalence could be the outcome of a very high mortality rate though with concurrent high incidence, which is by no means a desirable outcome. Demonstrating falling incidence is therefore the ultimate hope of all those engaged in HIV epidemiological surveillance, but it is technically very hard to do and it requires many years of follow-up. Thus it was not until the year 2000 before the very first evidence emerged of falling HIV incidence in Africa, at the Thirteenth International AIDS Conference in Durban (Mbulaiteye et al., 2000). Data from the MRC's general population cohort in Masaka showed statistically significant declining rates of HIV incidence between 1990 and 1999. Where 7.6 people in every thousand uninfected people were infected annually in 1990, the rate had fallen to 3.2 per thousand in 1998.

With this, Uganda's status as the African AIDS success story was sealed. The country's falling HIV prevalence rate became almost iconic, with the most widely circulated figures stating that national HIV prevalence had fallen from 30 percent early in the epidemic to 10 percent (see, for example, UAC, 2000:iii). In 2002, however, a London-based researcher, Justin Parkhurst, challenged in the *Lancet* the extent to which the figures were nationally representative. He did not claim that Uganda had not been successful in reducing HIV prevalence; rather, he suggested that the claims had been exaggerated through the use of "selective pieces of information, which have been falsely presented as representative of the nation as a whole" (Parkhurst, 2002:78). "The standard of proof for policy recommendations," he concluded, "seems to have been lowered to provide the international community with the African success story it wants, or even needs" (ibid.:80).

Parkhurst's intervention was not welcomed in Uganda. Captain Mike Mukula, the Health Minister, raged that "they don't believe that any country in Africa can do anything positive" (IRIN, 2002); and Parkhurst was characterized by several of my own respondents in Kampala as a foreign researcher whose approach I would do well not to emulate.

Did research contribute to Uganda's falling HIV infection rates?

The sort of evidence that would have been useful for policy makers and implementing agencies during this period is that which would have demonstrated the effectiveness or otherwise of particular HIV prevention strategies. By having an empirical basis, it would have helped to divide up limited funding between behavioral intervention channels such as peer education, school-based AIDS education, local video and drama shows, and nationwide poster and radio campaigns. It would also have been helpful to have an empirical basis for knowing which messages—for example, promoting abstinence, zero-grazing, or condom use—were most effective and acceptable, within which channels, and for which audiences.

However, very little such research had been conducted, so behavioral HIV prevention in Uganda and the rest of Africa continued to take place more or less in an evidence void. Perhaps the most comprehensive database detailing evaluations of African HIV behavioral interventions was run by the late John Hubley, formerly a Leeds-based health promotion specialist (Hubley, 2006). Hubley's database includes 41 peer-reviewed evaluations of African interventions up until the year 2002. These concern many different intervention strategies, including those targeting the general population or high-risk groups such as sex workers; those based in clinics and schools; and those using the mass media to put out their messages. Of these 41, 6 were conducted in Uganda (Schopper et al., 1995; Kaleeba et al., 1997; Kagimu et al., 1998; Shuey et al., 1999; Kipp et al., 2001; Kinsman et al., 2001).

At first sight, this may appear to be reasonably impressive. However, a closer analysis reveals a number of important holes in this body of evidence. First and foremost, the objective of all HIV prevention interventions is, obviously, the prevention of HIV—and yet only 2 of these 41 African studies have directly sought to verify that they have actually been preventing HIV transmission, by using HIV incidence as an outcome measure (Laga et al., 1994; Grosskurth et al., 1995). Furthermore, only one of these included a control group (Grosskurth et al., 1995), thereby permitting changes in the intervention group to be ascribed specifically to the intervention rather than to unknown external factors. And further still, although this study included a behavioral component, it was predominantly a clinical intervention that focused on the management of STDs. Thus, by 2002, the body of evidence did not include a single controlled evaluation of an African HIV behavioral intervention that used the marker that really matters—HIV incidence—as an outcome measure.

There are good reasons for this, not least the fact that conducting such rigorous evaluations is costly and technically complex. In mitigation, we should also remember that the Randomized Controlled Trial, by which such evaluations are conducted, does not have a monopoly as the only worthy methodological approach. Nonetheless, as Hubley points out in his database notes, much of the remaining evidence is of dubious quality, for a variety of reasons.

For example, all but half a dozen of the remaining 39 evaluations of African programs rely on Knowledge, Attitude, and Practice (KAP) surveys. The objective of these is to quantify people's knowledge about HIV and AIDS, in particular with respect to modes of transmission; their attitudes toward people living with AIDS and toward safer sex; and also to establish the proportions of people reporting—among other things— casual sex in the previous X months, or the proportion reporting condom use during such trysts. However, as suggested at the beginning of this chapter, such surveys are inherently subject to misreporting and bias, and provide only the shallowest of insights. Second, details of the intervention being evaluated—whether peer education or counseling or mass media campaigns—are frequently limited or missing entirely from the reports, which means that even if they were successful, nobody would be able to replicate them. Third, many of the evaluations include no baseline measurements and no details of sampling procedures, had very brief follow-up periods, or they do not provide the raw data on which their conclusions are drawn. Fourth, and very important from the point of view of evidence-based policy making, by no means all the studies reported success. Two of the six Ugandan studies, for example, reported either no or very limited effect of the intervention being evaluated (Kinsman et al., 2001; Kipp et al., 2001).

This critique shows that the literature on African behavioral interventions was of extremely varied quality, and that it would have been very difficult to take the findings collectively and argue that they show anything definitive. The possibility for developing any sort of evidence-based policy was therefore limited, while the conditions for moral, ideologically based policy making could hardly have been more perfect.

Within Uganda, it could be argued that the country's open policy to AIDS in some ways inadvertently facilitated this situation. The Uganda AIDS Commission published a National Research Needs Assessment for AIDS in 1993, which found that "a virtual explosion of activity" had taken place, during which "much of the research work has been ad hoc, without an overall coordinated plan, and with little effort of sustainability" (UAC, 1993:3). Furthermore, the trend noted above during the period 1986 to 1992—in which relatively little AIDS research was based in Africa, and even less was formulated and led by Africans—continued throughout the 1990s. As the Ugandan social scientist Christine Obbo complained, "the research agenda on AIDS in Uganda is determined by outsiders. The Ugandan doctors involved in AIDS research have become rubber stamp collaborators who cannot set the agenda because they are paid by someone else. Several doctors have said: 'This is the only way I can make a living to support my family.' 'This is the only way I can keep in touch with international researchers.' 'This is the only way I can travel, I do not want to be an isolated scientist.' 'We are a poor country; our hands are tied'" (Obbo, 1995:84). Given the effective absence of a usable evidence base for HIV prevention, one must conclude that either such work was not seen as relevant to the particular scientific interests of the expatriates who were setting the AIDS research agenda, or, given that a strong infrastructure is needed for such endeavors, they felt that conducting rigorous intervention evaluations was simply not feasible.

Such was the lack of firm evidence regarding HIV prevention in Uganda as well as in the rest of Africa that a group of international organizations felt obliged to issue a Statement of Belief, affirming their *belief* in the value and effectiveness of behavior change. The statement—by UNDP, the Salvation Army, Save the Children-UK, and the UK NGO AIDS Consortium—tried to sound confident, but its inevitable weakness illustrates the position that was being faced: "We believe that individuals and whole communities have the inherent capacity to change attitudes and behavior . . . We believe that behavior change is the most essential strategy in overcoming this HIV pandemic" (AIDS Analysis Africa, 1992:9).

UNAIDS was also suffering from desperation. One of my respondents, who had previously worked with the organization, decried the lack of evidence specifically in relation to voluntary HIV counseling and testing (VCT), but the principle applied equally to other prevention strategies: "As UNAIDS we emphasized the potential benefit [of VCT] for HIV prevention [in the mid-1990s] without solid evidence. This was the only thing we had in the armory. You sit back now and look at the evidence, and say we were desperate, but we had to do that. It was all we had." Such comments put an interesting perspective on the carefully crafted UNAIDS global update from June 1998, which includes a section entitled *Prevention Works* (UNAIDS, 1998:26). Since much of UNAIDS' work involves advocacy and awareness-raising, they were unlikely to suggest that prevention activities would *not* work; but the certainty of their statement belies the undeniably fragile basis on which it stood. Their own text conceded that "it is almost impossible to attribute changing behavior or low or falling rates of infection with HIV and other STDs to a single element of a prevention program" (ibid.:26); but it then went on to say that "all the evidence shows that prevention does work" (ibid.:26). The only evidence presented from all of Africa to support this claim came from Senegal, one of a small handful of sub-Saharan African countries that has consistently maintained very low levels of HIV prevalence.

Across the continent, therefore, enormous gaps remained in what was known about the effectiveness of HIV prevention strategies. In response to this, the MRC set up the Masaka Intervention Trial (MIT) in 1994, the first evaluation of an African community-based HIV behavioral intervention to use HIV incidence as its primary outcome measure. By using a hard biological outcome measure such as HIV incidence, the study could largely overcome the problems of desirability bias inherent in purely survey-based research; and, as such, it was hoped, could provide solid evidence of the effectiveness—or not—of the widely adopted approach to HIV prevention that it was evaluating. The MIT and the response to its findings, which were released in 2003, will be discussed in detail in Chapter 6.

(iii) 2002 to 2005—Money, Politics, and Mud

PEPFAR and the retrospective birth of ABC

"To meet a severe and urgent crisis abroad, tonight I propose the Emergency Plan for AIDS Relief—a work of mercy beyond all current international efforts to help the people of Africa . . . I ask the Congress to commit $15 billion over the next five years, including nearly $10 billion in new money, to turn the tide against AIDS in the most afflicted nations of Africa and the Caribbean" (Bush, 2003a). With these words, spoken on 28 January 2003, U.S. President George W. Bush opened an important new chapter in the global campaign against HIV and AIDS, as well as in the increasingly heated international and globalized discussion about how this campaign should be managed.

The U.S. President's Emergency Plan for AIDS Relief (PEPFAR) was—and remains—very ambitious. In its first five years (2003 to 2008), it aimed (i) to prevent 7 million new HIV infections; (ii) to bring 2 million

HIV-positive people onto antiretroviral therapy; and (iii) to provide "humane care" for 10 million HIV-infected individuals and AIDS orphans (Bush, 2003b). The legislation[18] that dictated how to spend the $15 billion requested by President Bush stipulated the following division:

1. Fifty-five percent for the treatment of people with AIDS;
2. Twenty percent for HIV prevention (of which at least 33 percent was to be spent on abstinence-until-marriage programs);
3. Fifteen percent for the palliative care of people with AIDS;
4. Ten percent for helping orphans and vulnerable children.

During the debates in Congress concerning how to allocate this $15 billion, the prevention component provoked particular controversy, with the arguments largely following the party political divide. Republicans generally argued in favor of abstinence-until-marriage programs while Democrats tended to support funding for condom promotion programs. Witnesses were invited to contribute, of whom one of the most crucial to the outcome was Uganda's First Lady, Janet Museveni. A devout Christian, she has consistently stood in firm opposition to the use of condoms, and especially so by young people. "Young people must be taught the virtues of abstinence, self control and postponement of pleasure, and sometimes sacrifice," she told an International Christian Conference on AIDS in February 2002 (*New Vision*, 2002b). "I am not comfortable," she added in October 2003, "with the thought that the [fate] of an entire continent could depend upon a thin piece of rubber" (*Monitor*, 2003).

With this well-defined advocacy position in mind, she flew to Washington, D.C., during the debates and presented a formal letter to Republican lawmakers stating that abstinence had been the key to Uganda's success (Epstein, 2007:187). Her lobbying, as well as that of various American Christian groups holding a similar position (see, for example, Dobson, 2003), helped to ensure that of the $3 billion that had been set aside for HIV prevention, at least 33 percent—or at least $1 billion—was to be used solely for abstinence-until-marriage programs. The basis of the policy included evidence provided to Congress that "abstinence until marriage has been shown to significantly reduce HIV infection rates on a continent otherwise ravaged by AIDS. Uganda once had the highest HIV infection rate in the world, but after launching an aggressive program prioritizing abstinence, the infection rate plummeted by as much as 70 percent, courtesy of a two-year delay in the onset of sexual activity among young people" (Dobson, 2003).

This sounds impressive, but it is epidemiologically incorrect. First, it is exaggerating to describe anything that took place in Uganda prior to

2004 as an "aggressive program prioritizing abstinence." In spite of international accolades (see, for example, Heckert and Baldo, 1998; Green, 2003a), AIDS and sex education in Ugandan schools—the most accessible setting for reaching large numbers of young people with messages about abstinence—has in fact historically been very limited. AIDS education was not included at all in the curriculum for Uganda's secondary schools throughout the 1990s (Kinsman et al., 1999:592; Hyde et al., 2002:vi), with a presentation given at the Ninth International Conference on AIDS and STD in Africa, held in Kampala in 1995, concluding that "sex education is virtually absent in [Ugandan] schools, or was limited purely to information on reproductive biology" (Bachengana, 1995). Subsequently, a life skills program was launched by the Ministry of Education and UNICEF (UNICEF, 1996), with the intention of "empowering girls and boys to be self-confident decision makers with the ability to delay sexual debut, negotiate safe sex and become responsible citizens" (Human Rights Watch, 2005). However, its evaluation three years later revealed that "none of the activities had succeeded in reaching the classroom" (Hyde et al., 2002:32).

Second, the delay in onset of sexual activity over the 1990s was not two years, but half that (Bessinger et al., 2003:12). And third, only a portion of the "plummeting infection rate" can be attributed to abstaining youth, since the fall in prevalence occurred throughout the entire adult population. The conclusions drawn by Janet Museveni and James Dobson were based on a selective use of evidence, and do not accurately represent what happened in Uganda.

When signing the legislation to initiate PEPFAR four months after his initial announcement, President Bush also used an adapted version of what had taken place in Uganda as the basis on which PEPFAR would approach prevention in all its recipient countries. "The nation of Uganda is pursuing a successful strategy of prevention," he said, "emphasizing abstinence and marital fidelity, as well as the responsible use of condoms to prevent HIV transmission. The results in Uganda have been remarkable. The AIDS infection rate has fallen sharply since 1990, and in some places the percentage of pregnant women with HIV has been cut in half. The Uganda plan is proving that major progress is possible" (Bush, 2003b). One of the key phrases used here referred to the "responsible use of condoms"; a model which, as defined by PEPFAR, included promoting condoms only for high-risk groups, such as sex workers and their clients; sexually active discordant couples (in which one partner is known to have HIV while the other remains HIV-negative); and substance abusers. Young people were not seen as appropriate targets for condom promotion (PEPFAR, 2005). Such specific targeting of condoms was never part of the Ugandan model, but nonetheless, Ugandan policy—or an *interpretation* of Ugandan policy—played a significant part in shaping and justifying a major U.S. foreign policy, which Bush himself described as "the largest single up-front commitment in history for an international public health initiative involving a specific disease" (White House, 2003b). Thereby, Ugandan policy, as seen through the ideological lens of the Bush administration, also subsequently affected the AIDS control strategies of all the early PEPFAR-recipient nations.

The "Uganda plan" being advocated by the U.S. administration was dubbed ABC: Abstain, Be faithful, or use a Condom. The term "ABC" was applied to Uganda by Americans, and had never actually been used in Uganda prior to 2002. It was in a sense, therefore, a retrospective and foreign definition of Uganda's AIDS control efforts since 1986. Since, at the individual level, A, B, and C represent the only three currently viable means for people to avoid the sexual transmission of HIV—and since Uganda has advocated for each of these strategies in different ways over the years—this is not in itself problematic. It does broadly represent what Uganda has done. A difficulty has arisen, however, in the relative emphasis given to the three components by advocates on each side of the ideological divide.

For example, former U.S. Secretary of State Colin Powell wrote to USAID missions in December 2002, requiring them to review all existing contracts with organizations involved in AIDS-related activities so as to ensure that they "reflect appropriately the policies of the Bush administration." He continued, telling them to promote an ABC policy, before adding that "empirical evidence shows that successful programs support a strong emphasis on campaigns that promote abstinence, faithfulness, and reduction of the number of partners" (*Boston Globe*, 2003:A1). With no mention of condoms, this amounted to an "empirically-based" ABC strategy with no C. As an American author complained, "U.S.-based social conservatives in and out of government—even as they pay homage to the ABC mantra—continue to confuse all of these issues. For them, ABC has become little more than an excuse and justification to promote their long-standing agenda regarding people's sexual behavior and the kind of sex education they should receive: A for all unmarried people, bolstered by advocacy of B, but, at least for the so-called general population, 'anything but C'" (Cohen, 2004:132). Indeed, some religious groups have recast ABC altogether during this rewriting of Ugandan history, with the C for Condoms being switched to C for Christ (Cushman, 2005).

On the other side of the divide was a wide array of actors also claiming evidence in support of their pro-condom position and adopting sometimes disingenuous wording to make their point. For example, a piece entitled *Closing the Condom Gap*, published by the prestigious Johns

Hopkins School of Public Health, includes the rather misleading statement that, "in Uganda condom use increased and HIV prevalence decreased following a national AIDS prevention and condom promotion effort" (Population Reports, 1999). While it is true that condom use increased and HIV incidence and prevalence simultaneously decreased, it is a major oversimplification to suggest that the former was primarily responsible for the latter: association is not the same as causation. As explained above, the number of condoms imported into the country annually could not possibly have counted for more than a handful of sex acts per couple per year; and while this would have contributed to a fall in incidence and prevalence, it was surely not the primary engine for change. It would appear that the pro-condom advocacy nature of the piece tempted the authors to imply a clear, if unjustified, link.

What really caused the fall in HIV incidence and prevalence?

Many of those involved in this debate have selected or interpreted evidence to suit a predetermined ideological position. But what does the evidence actually say? With the success of controlling HIV in Uganda, many researchers, both foreign and Ugandan, have become interested in trying to understand what had brought about the changes in the country. The epidemiology is not clear-cut, however, and, as explained by one of those involved in trying to unravel the story, the World Bank's David Wilson, "there is plenty in the data to bother everyone!" (USAID, 2002:1). An earlier study had suggested that risk behavior reduction—not mortality or migration—was primarily responsible for bringing down HIV prevalence in western Uganda (Kilian et al., 1999). The authors of this study did not, however, seek to ascertain the relative importance of particular individual-level behaviors—A, B, or C—in bringing about the changes. This was the question that defined the subsequent political debate over HIV prevention in Uganda.

In spite of the difficulties in interpreting the evidence, there is by now consensus among many international scientists that of the three components within the ABC strategy, B was of central importance in initially bringing down HIV incidence and prevalence in Uganda (Hogle et al., 2002; USAID, 2002; Green, 2003a; Shelton et al., 2004; Wilson, 2004; Stoneburner and Low-Beer, 2004). Much of the analysis for this early period relies on two nationwide survey datasets, collected in 1989 and 1995, the period in which the major turnaround in national prevalence took place. Known as Demographic and Health Surveys (DHS), these data suggested that Ugandans had reduced their number of non-regular (or higher-risk) sexual partners by as much as 60 percent during those years. As we have seen, condoms had not then been present in the country in anything like sufficient numbers to have had a significant population-level effect, and increases in reported abstinence were confined primarily to young, urban males. Rand Stoneburner of Cambridge University explained that "as the acceptance of partner reduction in Uganda occurred before interventions such as condom promotion, social marketing, and VCT[19] were implemented, the country's success appears to have taken root from the behavior changes motivated by this communication-based, community-level response to the epidemic" (USAID, 2002:3).

In other words, the turnaround in Uganda's HIV epidemic has been ascribed by many academics to the more austere end of the ABC spectrum—and especially to B—rather than to the more permissive, liberal C. One of the high-profile advocates of this interpretation of the evidence, Harvard University's Ted Green, has spoken of the problems inherent in this position, pointing out that "it would have been easier to promote the idea if Al Gore had been elected [U.S. President in 2000] rather than Bush, because nobody on the left would be suspicious that ABC was a Trojan Horse for abstinence-only groups on the right" (*Washington Times*, 2003). "In the present politically charged atmosphere," he added later, "it seems impossible to bring up evidence of this sort without being accused by someone of having an agenda that goes beyond AIDS" (Green, 2004).

One such accusing group was the New York–based organization Human Rights Watch (HRW), who charged that great behemoth—the U.S. government—with directing researchers such as Ted Green and his colleagues in their analysis of the Ugandan data. "Between 2002 and 2004," they wrote, "the U.S. government sponsored at least four studies which concluded that the drop in HIV prevalence in Uganda in the 1990s resulted from increased rates of abstinence and fidelity in Uganda during that period, as well as a concerted government effort to encourage these behavior changes. The aim of these studies was apparently to provide a scientific basis for current abstinence-until-marriage programs" (Human Rights Watch, 2005:68).

There are grounds for questioning the last sentence here, which could have the effect of discrediting the scientists involved in these studies. The objective of the HRW report was to challenge the increasing focus on abstinence-only programs in Uganda, as supported by the U.S. government; and its title, *The Less They Know, The Better*, makes clear the organization's position on the subject from the start. And while the report did include a robust critical assessment of the evidence in support of their position, it then went beyond the science by implying that since the Bush administration supported abstinence-based interventions, scientists who also argued along these lines did so, willingly or otherwise, under pressure from Washington. Few scientists would welcome such a charge, since it would call into question their scientific independence and integrity, which in turn would cast doubt on their findings. From this, one can begin to see what Ted Green meant when he talked about "agendas that go beyond AIDS."

A final word on the epidemiological complexity of HIV in Uganda is warranted here. The consistent conclusion among scientists about the preeminence of B has been jarred by a report from Rakai suggesting that sharp increases in condom use in the district over the period 1993 to 2004 were counterbalanced by decreases in both abstinence and faithfulness. The primary reason for falling HIV prevalence in the area, the authors concluded, was high mortality—people with AIDS dying, and thereby leaving the pool of infected individuals (Wawer et al., 2005). While this suggestion is not contradictory to the explanation above—it does not deny that B may have played an important role in the earliest years of the national response, prior to 1993—it does provide a more complex interpretation of what may have happened. There is indeed plenty in the data to worry everyone.

Thus the science may never produce a clear, unambiguous explanation for what happened in Uganda, but, as argued in an open letter published in the *Lancet* in November 2004—signed by over 100 individuals, including President Museveni—this chapter should now be closed. "The time has come," the letter argued, "to leave behind divisive polarization and to move forward together in designing and implementing evidence-based prevention programs to help reduce the millions of new infections occurring each year" (Halperin et al., 2004:1914).

Back in Uganda, the previous few months had seen an acrimonious resurgence of the condom debate, so this call came not a moment too soon.

A changing condom policy in Uganda: Under pressure from the United States?

During a keynote address at the Fifteenth International AIDS Conference in Bangkok in July 2004, President Museveni provoked a storm with a series of apparently contradictory comments about Uganda's HIV prevention policy. Museveni's words, as given below, should be seen in relation to the country's National Condom Policy and Strategy, which had almost certainly received his personal approval. Published just the month before the Bangkok conference, in June 2004, the condom policy states that "correct and consistent condom use shall be widely and openly promoted to all sexually active individuals as an effective means of preventing HIV/ STI transmission and as a family planning method" (ACP, 2004:8).

Museveni's first comments in Bangkok appeared to be a reiteration of the well-known Ugandan position: "Our approach [to HIV prevention] is gradual; abstinence, be faithful to each other, but if you can't, use a condom. It is a graduated process rather than another 'unit solution' approach . . . Let the condom be used for those who cannot abstain, those who cannot be faithful within marriage, or those who are estranged from their families for economic reasons. They may not have optimal sex according to our idea of sex; it may not be optimal, but it will be safe sex [and will] be better than dying."

But he then took an almost directly opposing position: "[The condom] is a good improvisation—I look at the condom as an improvisation, not as a solution, but an improvisation . . . People assume that all people in the world have sex in the same way . . . Condoms may be all right in some varieties [of sexual practices], but in other varieties it's quite a hindrance, and I am sure these Africans know what I am talking about [Laughter] . . . The prescription of condoms is not, in my opinion, the adequate solution to this problem in the end because in some cultures, sexual intercourse is so elaborate that condoms are a hindrance and therefore a frustration" (Kaiser Network, 2004).

Museveni may have been personally ambivalent about condoms for many years, but this rather mixed message—given in a high-profile speech and in his capacity as an esteemed international leader in the struggle against AIDS—generated significant debate both in Uganda and in Bangkok. The State Minister for Health, Dr. Alex Kamugisha, felt obliged to go on the record four days later to "clarify" what the President had actually meant. "The President pointed out several challenges regarding condom use especially in the Great Lakes region and in most of Africa, where they could be used inconsistently or inappropriately," Kamugisha said. "The President did not at any one time campaign against the use of condoms. On the contrary, he said denying condoms to people who need them would be condemning them to death. Condoms save lives if used correctly and consistently" (New Vision, 2004a).

In spite of the Minister's clarification, Museveni's anti-condom rhetoric resurfaced later in the year. In October 2004, he argued that "condoms are not the solution because there are certain sicknesses which cannot be stopped by condoms. This condomisation they are talking about is a recipe for disaster" (New Vision, 2004b). A similar position was put forward in November by the State Minister for Information, Dr. Nsaba Buturo, who said that, "we have erroneously given more prominence to condoms [than abstinence and faithfulness] and this is going to change. It is now going to be equal treatment . . . The strategy that has worked for Uganda is ABC but of late there has been a school of thought fiercely defending the position that it is the condom. They don't want anyone to talk about abstinence and faithfulness" (*New Vision*, 2004c). A change in rhetoric had emerged, suggesting a switch from the policy outlined in the recently published National Condom Policy and Strategy.

This change emerged during my fieldwork in late 2004, so I was able to ask relevant individuals what they thought had brought it about. Other background events were taking place at the time, such as the fact that 2004 saw Uganda receive her first tranche of PEPFAR money, to the tune of $91 million (PEPFAR, 2008). Most of my respondents appeared to believe that there was a direct connection between the incoming PEPFAR cash and the mixed policy messages, an indication of both Uganda's dependence on U.S. development aid and of the power of the United States to affect the domestic policies of foreign countries.

For example, a Resident District Commissioner—a political appointee of the President's own choosing—explained to me that, "initially, [Museveni] was reticent about condoms, then he embraced them, and now he's drawing away from them again. It's because of international pressure." A senior public health physician in Kampala felt similarly: "I wasn't in Bangkok, but the people I spoke to said that the Ugandans were holding their heads in their hands . . . To be sure, he has never been a favorite of condoms or premarital sex. But having watched him over the years, I've never heard him so openly denouncing them. That strong message may have come from his Republican friends in Washington. I think the Americans may have a strong impact."

Another public health physician held the same line. "My inclination is that the Bush money has changed the way we face the epidemic. It has encouraged the moralists to speak with a louder voice, and to kill the condom aspect. Bangkok was when he made it public to the outside world, but even before that he had said it here. Two or three years ago, he gave a talk and he lambasted the condom." This comment provides some confirmation of the views of the Masaka Bishop, as given above, who believed that condom promotion was encouraged by foreign donors in Uganda during the 1990s, with the caveat that "either you accept the condoms, or we stop the aid." There is a clear suggestion here that the direction of the international political wind largely dictates the direction of HIV prevention practices in Uganda.

However, not all my respondents felt that U.S. pressure was behind the changes. A journalist working with the government-backed *New Vision* newspaper explained that "the way I interpret [what Museveni said in

Bangkok] is that he didn't say anything new; he has never really been an advocate of condoms. It's just that he was in a different forum. He was just advocating for ABC, as usual. Maybe it pleased President Bush, but it was the same position he's always had. He couldn't have taken that position to please Bush."

An editorial for the same newspaper argued similarly: "The most disheartening fact was for [Museveni's critics] to insinuate that he was seeking cheap favors from U.S. President George Bush. To the critics of the President's downplaying of condoms, he is ostensibly trying to hang on Bush's coat tails since the U.S. President too is no fan of condoms. In return, the Ugandan leader supposedly collects dollar crumbs from the American high table. Of course, the peddlers of this desperate argument pretend not to know that President Museveni was deep in the anti-HIV/AIDS trenches long before baby Bush got out of political diapers" (*New Vision*, 2004d).

Clear divisions had therefore emerged in 2004 within Uganda over the direction of the country's condom policy. In an unfortunate further development, the confusion was exacerbated late in the year by a Ministry of Health decision to withdraw tens of millions of Chinese-manufactured condoms, known as *Engabo*,[20] from government clinics and distributors across the country. Customers had complained of a bad sulfurous smell, and post-shipment tests had also revealed substandard latex with many holes (Bass, 2005). Given the simultaneous change in Uganda's de facto condom policy, the timing could hardly have been worse for the Ministry of Health, which holds a pro-condom position. I was present at a public meeting in November 2004, at which Dr. Elizabeth Madraa, then head of the Ministry's ACP, tried to rectify the public's perception of what had happened. "All the condoms we bring [into Uganda] are really good condoms," she said. "But we are rectifying that [problem with Engabo], and we make sure that the condoms which we give out are quality condoms. We are really concerned about the quality, and we are sorry about the mishap." In spite of Madraa's pleas, there were suggestions among some members of the public that this was Museveni's way of withdrawing support for the condom via the back door (IRIN, 2006). Museveni's political position, they suggested, had been manifested via a faked technical problem with the Chinese condom manufacturers.

Uganda's condom shortage remained unresolved for some time, creating serious ongoing problems for HIV prevention programs throughout the country. Indeed, the total number of condoms sold and distributed for free in the country fell from 90 million in 2003 to 39 million in 2004 (Wabwire-Mangen et al., 2009:23). However, the crisis also turned into a political football, with Stephen Lewis, the UN's Special Envoy on AIDS in

Africa, attributing the shortage directly to U.S. policies: "There is no doubt in my mind that the condom crisis in Uganda is being driven by [U.S. programs]," Lewis said. "Over the last eight to ten months, there's been a very significant decline in the use of condoms, significantly orchestrated by the policies of the [U.S.] government" (*Monitor*, 2005). It is not possible to say with any certainty whether or not the United States was really behind Uganda's condom shortage. But Mr. Lewis' comments once again underscore the strength of feeling that existed on both sides of the debate, feelings that were defined above all by ideology rather than by evidence.

Discussion

This detailed historical review has shown that the major decisions during the first 15 years or so of behavioral HIV prevention in Uganda were based primarily on educated hunches, pragmatism in the face of limited alternatives, and a clear understanding of what could feasibly be attempted. None of what was done in those years was evidence-based in the sense that any given strategy—first zero-grazing and then an increasingly liberal national condom promotion strategy—had been scientifically shown to be effective. But Uganda was lucky, and collectively the approach worked, with HIV prevalence peaking in the early 1990s, and then falling steadily throughout the decade.

This success in bringing down prevalence rates stimulated great interest from the year 2002 onwards, when huge sums of money were becoming available for combating AIDS in Africa through such funding mechanisms as President Bush's PEPFAR. Impetus was thus created for bringing evidence onto center stage for the first time. With Uganda's unique success in reducing its HIV burden over the 1990s, PEPFAR administrators looked to supporting evidence from the country to justify the HIV prevention policies that they wanted to develop.

It was not, however, the actual Ugandan approach to HIV prevention that was adopted as the PEPFAR model for HIV prevention. Rather, it was an *interpretation* of Uganda's experience that was presented to the world by President Bush as the "Uganda Plan." This focused considerably more on abstinence and considerably less on condoms than was justified by the limited data that existed on the subject. The retrospective interpretation of past events was then used as the template on which U.S.-funded HIV prevention programs were to be run in all 15 PEPFAR-recipient countries, including Uganda. Thus a rewriting of Uganda's historical approach to HIV prevention—the ABC policy—was reflected back onto a willing and receptive Uganda via Washington, and presented as if it had been Uganda's idea in the first place.

Ironically, one could argue that Uganda's long-standing open AIDS policy—which provided an umbrella for all the events described in this chapter—partially facilitated this outcome. AIDS research in Uganda has always been driven primarily by non-Ugandan actors and interests, to the point that it was already recognized in 1993 that the explosion in research activity in the country was uncoordinated and ad hoc. Evaluations of complex behavioral interventions were simply not the priority of Western-based scientists, who were more interested in simply understanding the scale of the epidemic. Their research focus was manifested through the "numbing sero-epidemiologies" mentioned in the text, which, the rationale ran, would be invaluable as advocacy material. If HIV prevalence was shown to be high, it was felt that donors would be more sympathetic to requests for increases in funding for AIDS prevention and care services. This meant, however, that very little research had focused on evaluating HIV prevention interventions, which meant in turn that when the advocacy finally bore fruit in the form of the PEPFAR billions, there was almost nothing concrete in terms of demonstrably effective strategies on which to base decisions about how to spend all the money. Thus, conditions were ripe for a value-based decision making process.

It was within this evidence void that a strategic coalition of Ugandan and American Christian groups successfully lobbied the U.S. Congress to ensure that $1 billion would be set aside for abstinence-only HIV prevention programs in PEPFAR-recipient countries. Uganda's First Lady, Janet Museveni, was a key member of this evangelical coalition. As described in Chapter 2, Moynihan explains how advocate groups can help bring about policy changes, by drawing together three components: social movement, knowledge generation, and political activity. Together, he argues, these can become "the triangle that moves the [policy] mountain" (Moynihan, 2004:18). In this case, the three components were as follows:

1. *Social movement*: Christian evangelicals—both Ugandan and American—constituted the social movement behind the drive for a particular interpretation of ABC, which focused on a "moral" approach to HIV prevention.
2. *Knowledge generation*: A limited amount of knowledge had been generated in Uganda about the most effective means of preventing HIV, and there were ambiguities within the body of evidence. The Christian evangelical social movement collectively selected the evidence that supported its case for a moral agenda.
3. *Political activity*: When Congressional debates were underway to discuss how the PEPFAR pot should be split up, Janet Museveni travelled to Washington, D.C., and joined her American ideological

colleagues in their lobbying work. Her status as the First Lady of Uganda—*the* African AIDS success story—and as wife of *the* African AIDS leader lent her message enormous credibility and authority.

An interesting contrast can be drawn between this process and that which arose out of the Mwanza trial (Grosskurth et al., 1995), conducted in neighboring Tanzania. The Mwanza trial (described in more detail in Chapter 6) was the first African study to demonstrate unequivocally that a given approach to HIV prevention could work. This approach was clinic-based syndromic STD management, and the study's success stimulated important policy changes for STD management and HIV prevention throughout Africa (Philpott et al., 2002). Walt et al. (2003) describe how the Mwanza results went through a series of "iterative loops" as the findings became incorporated into international policy. A "bottom-up, research-oriented" loop from Tanzania fed into a process of policy standardization and formulation at the international level, which included such international organizations as the WHO, the World Bank, and the European Commission. This was then followed by a "top-down, marketing-oriented" loop, during which the new, agreed policy of promoting syndromic STD management was marketed and promoted throughout Africa. Through this process, "complex, context-specific policies [were] re-packaged into simplified guidelines for global best practice" (Walt et al. 2003:3).

A similar three-stage process took place with Uganda's ABC policy, though with important differences at each stage. The first, bottom-up stage involved the country's successful HIV prevention campaign, up until around 2000. Unlike Mwanza, however, this was a hunch-based success, not one based on a scientific approach. The second stage involved taking the Ugandan experience out of Uganda, and repackaging it in Washington. Unlike Mwanza, this repackaging was fuelled not by evidence but by a clearly defined ideological agenda. The third stage involved the marketing and promotion of this repackaged Ugandan experience throughout Africa by PEPFAR. Unlike syndromic STD management, which was promoted by a wide-ranging partnership of international public health professionals, ABC became the domain of a single, powerful donor. This final stage demonstrates the extent to which the Americans needed their Ugandan partners, just as the Ugandans needed the Americans, in pursuing their respective ideological and political agendas. The money and the ostensible power may have been American, but the initial, all-important basis for the idea was Ugandan.

This is therefore not the first instance of a looped international health policy transfer. The central difference, however, is that the coalition that won the interpretative battle of what had happened in Uganda—the Christian evangelists—did so on the basis of a highly contested analysis of the evidence. The result was that a significant portion of PEPFAR's early, Africa-wide HIV prevention policy was based on only the most questionable of evidence foundations.

This conclusion is not merely of academic interest—it has also had important implications for the people of Uganda. The country was undoubtedly successful in its HIV prevention campaign throughout the 1990s and very early 2000s, but continued success can never be taken for granted. Indeed, just as the first signs of falling incidence were observed in Masaka (Mbulaiteye et al., 2000), the very first signs of a possible resurgence in the epidemic were also noted there (Shafer and Opio, 2006). A subsequent report has warned of a national-level shift toward more risk-taking behaviors, including an increase in multiple sexual partnerships and nonspousal sex, and a decrease in condom use in nonspousal sex among men (Opio et al., 2008). It is clear that the national HIV prevention strategy now needs reinvigoration and new ideas.

This chapter has shown that behavioral HIV prevention in Uganda has never been truly evidence-based. But there *is* now evidence—as presented in a comprehensive review from the Uganda AIDS Commission, that includes both the epidemiology of HIV infection and HIV prevention activities throughout the country—that "the greatest need for HIV prevention exists among persons with multiple partners" (Wabwire-Mangen et al., 2009:32). While this undoubtedly presents a major challenge, it also presents an excellent opportunity for developing innovative approaches to reduce new infections.

Anthropologist Robert Thornton has sketched out a convincing proposal for such an approach, which he calls *One, One, One* (Thornton, 2008). *One, One, One* expands the individualistic perspective for HIV prevention that has been the hallmark of ABC, to include the sexual network of which individuals are a part. The approach encourages people to stick with *one* partner at a time (thereby reducing the number of links in their sexual network); to wait *one* month before starting sex with a new partner (since people are particularly infectious during their first month of HIV infection); and to choose their sexual partner from within *one* locale (since this will reduce the geographical scale of the network). A partial version of this is currently being run by the Uganda Health Marketing Group, whose nationwide *One Love* campaign slogan calls for people to "get off the sexual network" and stick to one partner. Currently, however, there are no significant Ugandan interventions addressing the other two *Ones*.

It makes great sense to focus on the sexual network as a means of HIV prevention in Uganda's current epidemiological conditions. *One, One, One* does, however, remain only in concept form, which means that a number of important questions still need to be addressed:

1. How, exactly, should its HIV prevention messages be formulated?
2. Which target populations should these messages focus on?
3. How and through which channels should the messages be put forward?
4. What would be the best means of conducting and evaluating a pilot *One, One, One* intervention?

Donors, international agencies, and the Ugandan government should all actively support efforts to answer these questions, and—if the pilot is successful—to embark on a scaled-up *One, One, One* intervention. Thornton himself has argued that behavioural HIV prevention has become "fossilised" around ABC (Thornton, 2008:221); this is an opportunity to bring it back to life.

5

Overcoming Resistance: Big Men and the Scale-Up of Antiretroviral Therapy Provision

Introduction

The rapid emergence across the globe of large-scale antiretroviral therapy (ART) programs for people living with AIDS has been nothing short of a revolution. In the space of just four years, the number of people in low- and middle-income countries receiving this life-saving treatment increased fivefold, from 240,000 in 2001 to 1.3 million at the end of 2005 (WHO, 2006a). By December 2008, the number had expanded yet further, to over 4 million, of whom around 3 million were in sub-Saharan Africa (WHO, 2009a).

Such figures would have been unthinkable at the turn of the millennium; but where AIDS was once effectively a sentence of death for people in Africa, it has become—for many, if not for all—a chronic, manageable condition. In 2005, a global target of universal access for all those in need of ART was set by the G8 group of industrialized nations, to be reached by 2010 (G8, 2005); and while it is clear that the target will not now be met—around 58 percent of the 9.5 million people in need of treatment were still not receiving it at the end of 2008 (WHO, 2009a)—ART has nonetheless become a permanent and central feature of the global AIDS control landscape.

How did this revolution come about? What were the processes and influences that contributed, and to what extent did research play a role? Why were some people so concerned about large-scale ART programs, and what problems have already been faced that might act as a prelude for the future? These are the questions addressed in this chapter, which charts the evolution of ART provision up to and including 2005, at all three levels—locally, in Masaka; in Uganda as a whole; and also globally. The chapter moves through the three levels as it moves across time, thereby demonstrating the interconnected and interdependent nature of the entire phenomenon.

One of the main themes to emerge is the resistance that was faced by those seeking to expand ART provision. There were many different reasons for this resistance, and these varied between levels. But the rapid scale-up of ART provision globally and in Uganda during the early- and mid-2000s ultimately took place because of the collective determination of advocacy coalitions to force through their will in spite of the opposition they faced. Advocacy coalitions are groups of "people from a variety of positions . . . who share a particular belief system—that is, a set of basic values, casual assumptions, and problem perceptions—and who show a non-trivial degree of co-ordinated activity over time" (Sabatier, 1993:25). In this case, the coalitions were led by individuals working in the political and financial spheres at each level. They are described here as Big Men—there were very few women involved at the most senior levels—and they were determined to put in place what they believed to be an essential humanitarian response to the catastrophic African AIDS epidemic.

The discussion in this chapter focuses on ART provision for HIV-positive adults, and is not concerned with use of the drugs for the prevention of mother-to-child HIV transmission (PMTCT).

Toward ART Provision in Uganda (1987–2001)

The treatment of AIDS in Uganda did not start with ART. The world's first antiretroviral drug (ARV)—zidovudine or AZT—was approved by the U.S. Food and Drug Administration for use against HIV in March 1987; and at a cost of around $10,000 per year, it was effectively accessible only to patients in wealthy Western countries. Ugandans living with AIDS at that time had to rely on more basic approaches to treatment, which focused on the treatment of the diverse opportunistic infections (OIs) brought about by HIV-related immunosuppression. At its best, this method could provide some relief, but care in Uganda during the 1980s was still very basic. In the words of an experienced counselor, "[P]eople don't die so miserably nowadays. They used to have such terrible diarrhea so that you wondered if the HIV even destroyed their intestines. And the skin was so bad, peeling off. You could enter a room with an AIDS patient, and it was smelling terribly. But now treatment and counseling have improved things so much." The treatment of OIs was difficult and rarely effective over the longer term, and patients would suffer from one infection after another until they eventually and inevitably succumbed.

Two groundbreaking institutions emerged in Masaka during the late 1980s, to provide care for people living with AIDS: Kitovu hospital's mobile care unit, and The AIDS Support Organisation (TASO). Kitovu Mobile was established to complement the services of the 220-bed Kitovu mission hospital. During some periods, over 90 percent of patients admitted to the medical wards were suffering from AIDS-related conditions (Kitovu, 1993:4), and this drained the already-limited resources from other important areas. Something entirely separate was necessary to deal exclusively with AIDS patients, but setting up the new unit was not easy. "It was very difficult to get staff to work for me," founder and former Director Sister Ursula Sharpe explained. "And if a patient died, we were ostracized. But if they lived for a while, then people came and said, here's my brother, take care of him too. I made a decision to go only to the most inaccessible places where people had no health care, and we would only deal with AIDS. If we'd not stuck to that, then we'd always have been dealing with malaria instead. There were lots of obstacles: some of the witchdoctors opposed us because we were taking away business from them. And it was impossible to get a nurse to talk about HIV prevention, because immediately they did, then people said 'they're looking for sex.'" In spite of the difficulties, a total of 9,800 individual patients had been seen by Kitovu Mobile staff in the six years up to 1993; by when 3,100 were known to have died (Kitovu, 1994:3).

The second institution, TASO, also took a community-based approach to care, through the provision of counseling, information, medical and nursing care, as well as material assistance for people with AIDS and their families (Kalibala and Kaleeba, 1989). TASO's main message was for clients to "live positively," both in terms of trying to lead a healthy lifestyle and also by maintaining a positive mental and emotional outlook. The first TASO branch opened in Kampala in 1987, with the second opening in the old measles ward of Masaka's government hospital in November 1988. Four years after its founding, the organization was serving 6,000 people out of the two branches (Kaleeba et al., 1991). It was not, however, always easy to attract patients. A counselor who worked in the Masaka office in the late 1980s spoke of the problem of patients presenting too late. Many of their clients in the early days came only "once the witchdoctor had exhausted their pocket, and then they referred them to us. For example, they would say they have cured the diarrhea, but the patient now needs the hospital so that the scars in the stomach can be healed by the western medicine. So we decided to go out into the community and get people to come in before they wasted all their money on the witchdoctors."

In broad terms, therefore, the framework in Masaka for treating people with AIDS at this time was limited to "witchdoctors," and Kitovu Mobile or TASO.[1] No doubt, the health workers would have given a great deal to be able to provide their patients with the only ARV then available—AZT—had it been affordable. By contrast to the treatment of OIs as explained above, ARVs attack HIV directly by inhibiting viral replication, thereby reducing its destructive impact on the immune system. ARVs do not provide a cure, but this approach to treatment is nonetheless far more likely to bring about a longer-term reprieve from disease than mere management of OIs. With regard to AZT, however, it was quickly recognized that HIV's extraordinary rate of replication permitted it to overwhelm the drug's line of attack by evolving resistance to it. As a Ugandan Ministry of Health information paper explained in 1989, "life expectancy can be increased for one year to two years," but the patient would eventually die anyway (MoH, 1989:10).

Given AZT's cost and its relative lack of effectiveness, there was a great deal of skepticism about whether or not ARVs would ever be viable in Uganda. A former volunteer expatriate who worked in Masaka from 1988 to 1990 had thought it would be "a thousand years" before anything like that came to Uganda. Dr. Peter Mugyenyi, Uganda's first ART-providing pioneer, concurred, describing at the Uganda Medical Association's annual conference in December 2004, how "expert opinion" in the mid-late 1990s had held that an advanced version of ART—triple therapy—would prove to be "impossible" to use in Africa. Laboratory breakthroughs had led in 1996 to the introduction of triple therapy, a treatment approach that includes a cocktail of three different classes of ARVs.[2] By attacking three different types of enzymes necessary for viral replication, triple therapy significantly slows down the development of drug resistance. Also known as Highly Active AntiRetroviral Therapy (HAART), triple therapy remains the standard treatment for AIDS to this day.

There may have been consensus among many public health experts that ART in Africa would prove to be not viable, but Dr. Mugyenyi had in fact been providing the drugs in various formulations since 1991, at the Joint Clinical Research Centre (JCRC) in Kampala, a specialist AIDS treatment center that he had founded with the Ministries of Defence, Health, and Education. At this stage, ART remained accessible only to the privileged few Ugandans who could pay, and also to those lucky patients who found themselves eligible for participation in research projects.

Peter Mugyenyi explained the reasons for this in an e-mail he wrote to me in early 2005:

There were absolutely no donors willing to consider any support for ART until just recently. We initially provided for those who could afford the cost, and took steps to increase access by persuading employers and private sponsors to support treatment for the poor. From 1992 we had regular and incremental importation of drugs as demand and access increased. By 1996 when HAART became available we were treating over 1,000 patients with the same drugs as were then being used in USA.

Being in a research centre helped a great deal. Simply put, without a research setup we probably would have found it much more difficult to succeed. In research we worked with international experts who, though they never participated in any aspect of provision of ART or establishment of the program, assisted me initially in identifying sources of the drugs and helped in initial importation. Then we took over completely and regularly carried out drugs cost intelligence to access cheaper sources. The drugs initially flowed in without much problems because, as a research centre we could get in unlicensed drugs.

Through this work, Mugyenyi and his colleagues proved the experts wrong: ARV provision *was* feasible in Uganda. But since JCRC was providing the drugs at a significant cost to most of their patients, the great majority of Ugandans who needed them could not afford them. With around 1,000 patients on therapy in 1996, JCRC was meeting 1 percent or less of total national demand.[3]

Prices may have remained high, but at least the treatment now available—HAART—was relatively effective. On this basis, and with the viability of provision in Uganda established at JCRC, the Ugandan government took an important step toward expanding access to ART. On 5 November 1997, the Minister of Health, Crispus Kiyonga, announced that Uganda would participate in a four-country pilot project run by UNAIDS, called the Drug Access Initiative (DAI). "Uganda and other poor countries have argued that we should be assisted so that these drugs can reach those in need," the Minister said. "The pilot phase will be aimed at developing new strategies for removing obstacles to improved HIV/AIDS-related health care" (*New Vision*, 1997c).

The DAI would constitute the "first experiences of organized ARV delivery in Africa" (Katzenstein et al., 2003:S2), with the stated objective of "setting up the necessary infrastructure and systems to increase access to HIV-related drugs[4] on a small but sustainable scale" (ibid.:S1). Five centers were accredited in Uganda to act as providers when the project was launched in August 1998, all of which were in Kampala; and even though the drugs were subsidized and prices continued to fall, patients still had to pay a large monthly sum. Triple therapy had cost 1.7 million shillings per month (about $1,000) when it first appeared on the market in 1996, a cost that had fallen to 900,000 shillings (about $500) by 1999 (*Monitor*, 2001).

The needs of all Uganda's AIDS patients would never be met under such conditions—equitable provision to the general population remained a distant dream—but it still represented considerable progress. As the Uganda AIDS Commission commented, "even a journey of a thousand miles must start with one step" (UAC, 1997:14). And indeed, by 2001— when the DAI pilot project was transformed by UNAIDS into a wider Accelerated Access Initiative—Uganda had ten ARV-providing centers in operation, and drug costs to patients had fallen yet further. Depending on the regimen a patient was prescribed, monthly charges now ranged from 155,000 Uganda shillings (about $90) to 870,000 Uganda shillings (about $500) (IPPPH, 2003:34). The establishment of this preferential pricing system, and the associated move toward a sustainable program, was one of the DAI's major accomplishments.

The DAI was not, however, an unqualified success. Although its evaluation concluded that the "pilot programme successfully expanded access to antiretroviral drugs in Uganda" (Weidle et al., 2002:34), clinical and laboratory data presented for 476 of the 912 patients who took part in the project showed a number of problems with this model of provision. These were concerned primarily with the cost of the drugs. Clinical outcomes were compromised for the 49 percent of patients who could not afford the full triple therapy of three complementary ARVs, opting instead for a cheaper and less effective regimen with just two drugs. Furthermore, 33 percent of those who did not manage to adhere to their regimens as prescribed cited financial constraints as the reason. They were simply unable to pay for the drugs. The result of the difficulties faced in maintaining optimal adherence to an effective regimen was that resistance developed to at least one of the ARVs in 65 percent of the patients (ibid.:38). A method would have to be found to provide the drugs at no cost to patients; otherwise, ART in Uganda would remain no more than an expensive delay on their inexorable path to the grave.

In spite of these problems, the DAI had a significant impact on the international policy landscape, by highlighting what could be achieved as well as the difficulties that would inevitably be faced by such programs (IPPPH, 2003:36). The situation internationally was also profoundly affected by the decision early in 2001, of India's leading drug company, Cipla, to produce cut-price generic versions of the expensive, branded ARVs. As a generic drug, no patent payment would be due to the company that originally developed it, which meant that instead of costing $350 per month, triple therapy could now cost as little as $350 per *year* (*Guardian*, 2001).

Suddenly, large-scale ARV provision became a realistic goal even for poor African countries and, by June 2002, 80 countries had expressed interest in participating in the DAI's successor project, the Accelerated Access Initiative. Thirty-nine of these had already developed plans of action; 22 countries had entered negotiations with pharmaceutical companies; and 19 had successful UN-brokered supply agreements for ARVs (IPPPH, 2003:76). In other words, the work of the DAI along with the fall in drug prices contributed to a huge increase in demand for ARVs throughout the developing world. ARV provision was now demonstrably feasible in Africa and, with donor assistance, it was realistic to begin to think of national programs that were both sustainable and equitable.

But the authorities in Uganda remained unconvinced specifically about the sustainability of any large-scale ART operation, and were consequently very reluctant to permit the importation of generic ARVs when they came onto the market. It took the politically astute maneuverings of JCRC's Peter Mugyenyi to force the issue. "The problem arose [in 2001]," he explained, "when the demand for ART became huge and we faced a moral dilemma. So many poor patients were then besieging JCRC in desperate need of the life saving drugs! I do not know about the others, but to me it was just unbearable. I could not just stand by and do nothing about the appalling situation, as almost all the patients came to see me personally. I and only I took the decision to import generics. I couldn't even risk involving others as it would have been most unwise. I knew very well that the drugs would be impounded and that I was breaking the NDA[5] statute. Indeed, I planned to precipitate a crisis so that the catastrophe and tragedy of patients could come in acute focus and be addressed. I was also aware that this could land me in jail and was prepared for that, if only it could help speed up access and save some lives. I am not a confrontational person and very much hate to go against the law but I felt I had no alternative and reasonably there was none. When the drugs arrived at the airport without import licence or any kind of prior authorisation, they were, consistent with my expectation, impounded. A crisis was precipitated, and NDA wanted me punitively punished, but what followed is now well known. In brief, thousands, now in excess of 20,000, are alive because of this move."

A journalist at the *New Vision* newspaper explained further how Mugyenyi worked to change the NDA's provisional import license into a more enduring legal arrangement. "Mugyenyi was playing games with the NDA and the government. He said I've imported the drugs, they cost little, but you [the government] have impounded them and people continue to die. Finally the government let the drugs through, and Mugyenyi phoned me and said they have let them through. This was supposed to be a one-off, but then he said these people need to continue taking the drugs, so he imported another consignment. And that is how he broke the ground for ARVs to come into Uganda."

It was therefore the financial advantages of importing generic ARVs that inspired a determined Peter Mugyenyi to challenge the political and legal status quo, and that subsequently set the scene for the large-scale provision of ART in Uganda.

Doubts about Global ART Scale-Up

Even after securing permission to import generic ARVs, few Ugandans could afford the $350 annual cost of the drugs, and certainly the government did not have the financial capacity to provide any sort of subsidy for them. However, a spark of international interest was emerging, stimulated partially by the Clinton administration's description of AIDS as a threat to U.S. national security and to global stability (*Independent*, 2000); and partially by the fall in price of ARVs, which, for the first time, created conditions whereby the global humanitarian disaster of AIDS might be comprehensively addressed. Moves were therefore soon afoot to establish major funding agencies for ART provision in developing countries. Consequently, where the activists at the Geneva (1998) and Durban (2000) International AIDS Conferences had been saying, "this *must* be done," the mantra was now "this *can* be done." An unstoppable momentum was building to scale up ART provision throughout the developing world.

Given the long-standing role of the International AIDS Conferences in highlighting the dominant issues of the day, it was fitting that the next Conference, held in July 2002 in Barcelona, should have been the venue at which an ambitious goal for global ART scale-up was presented. Dr. Gro Harlem Brundtland, WHO Director General, announced in a keynote address that, "we are aiming for three million people world-wide to be able to access ARVs by 2005" (WHO, 2002a)—a vision that became known as '3 by 5' when it was formally launched in September 2003 by her successor, Dr. Lee Jong-wook. Given the recognition that ART was now potentially feasible in developing countries, '3 by 5' was intended to create global leadership and a political framework within which countries and donors would seek to scale up provision, and to turn the potential into a reality.

The two major donors that effectively legitimized this powerful political act were the Global Fund to Fight AIDS, Tuberculosis and Malaria (GFATM) and the U.S. President's Emergency Plan for AIDS Relief (PEPFAR). Inspired by a call in May 2001 from UN Secretary General, Kofi Annan, the Global Fund had started work in January 2002. Annan's idea was for a "war chest" of between 7 and 10 billion dollars to be spent annually on a global campaign against AIDS. Ensuring that care and treatment is within reach of all was, he said, a "personal priority" for him (Ferriman, 2001:1082). Subsequently, in January 2003 came George W Bush's announcement of his intention to establish PEPFAR, as described in Chapter 4. PEPFAR legislation required that 55 percent of the fund's $15 billion—or $8.25 billion—would be spent on treating people with AIDS between 2003 and 2008, of which 75 percent, or nearly $6.2 billion, would be spent on the purchase and distribution of ARVs (Avert, 2006). Thus, within the space of two years, a political and financial framework had been established for the global scale-up of ART provision, and there remained no obstacle to any developing country applying for and accessing the necessary funds for their own national program.

But not everyone thought that this move toward rapid treatment scale-up in the developing world was a good idea. I attended a conference held in Ottawa by the International Society for Sexually Transmitted Diseases Research in July 2003, a biannual scientific meeting to discuss biomedical, behavioral, and social aspects of STDs, including HIV. The meeting took place at a key moment in the history of ART scale-up, just before '3 by 5' was formally launched, but just after the establishment of the major funding bodies such as PEPFAR and the Global Fund. ART scale-up was therefore very much on people's minds.

One of the keynote speeches was given by Mark Wainberg, a Canadian molecular biologist and former President of the International AIDS Society, the group that organizes the International AIDS Conferences. He argued passionately that there was "no reason" not to scale up ART provision, and "no justification" for saying that ARV scale-up in Africa will lead to drug resistant virus. The danger of wide-scale resistance developing to ARVs was one of the arguments made by those urging caution in relation to scale-up, as explained later in this chapter. But Wainberg's rationale was that African patients are highly motivated to adhere to their drug regimens—perhaps more so than many Western patients—since the implications of the death of the family breadwinner are inevitably that much more critical in a society that lives close to the margins of survival. "There is no longer anyone else to whom the buck can be passed, but the politicians," he asserted (Wainberg, 2003).

I spoke with a number of conference delegates—all with long-standing experience of AIDS research in Africa—about Wainberg's speech, and met with universal skepticism about his view. A Professor of International Health told me that he "strongly disagreed" with his comments about adherence in Africa for ARVs not being a problem, and that he had been "playing to the gallery." If this had been one of the International AIDS Conferences, the Professor said, Wainberg would have been applauded by the activists—but not in this scientific setting. A Professor of Medical

Microbiology agreed, explaining that, "Mark has never lived or worked in Africa. He's a very concerned kind of person, an extremely smart guy, an eloquent speaker, but I don't think he understands the reality of Africa."

A senior clinical scientist argued similarly: "This man was head of the IAS.[6] I don't know, his perceptions of what it's really going to be like getting ARVs into developing countries, he's so far off the map. But he's obviously been to a lot of these International AIDS Conferences where you can make emotional statements like that about ARVs, and everyone gets up and cheers. And he kept pausing, and playing up to the crowd, but everyone was rolling their eyes."

Why were these experienced Western scientists so skeptical about the humanitarian position being upheld by Wainberg and the other advocates of ART scale-up? Three major points emerged during discussions with my respondents at the Ottawa conference and elsewhere, each of which has potentially enormous public health implications. The points included (i) the risk that the growing focus on ART would dilute or supersede HIV prevention activities; (ii) the risk that resistant virus would be generated through sub-optimal adherence to ARV drug regimens, thereby rendering treatment ineffective; and (iii) doubts over ART program sustainability. But to each of these concerns, the ART advocates had a response.

(i) The risk to HIV prevention

Concerns about the possible negative impact of treatment on prevention had been voiced long before wide-scale ART became a feasible option for Africa. As far back as 1991, there had been arguments suggesting that since ARVs will help people with AIDS to live longer, patients will have more time and opportunity to spread the disease, thus undermining prevention efforts (WorldAIDS, 1991:4). Former WHO Director General Hiroshi Nakajima subsequently warned in May 1997—shortly after HAART had emerged as an effective treatment for AIDS—that "the wave of optimism that has enveloped the international AIDS community in relation to the new therapies must not lead policy makers to abandon their commitment to essential long-term activities such as prevention programmes" (New Vision, 1997d). A Lancet article had also argued that HIV prevention was as much as 28 times more cost-effective than treatment, and that funding HAART at the expense of prevention would result in "greater loss of life" (Marseille et al., 2002:1851).

There were also concerns about an increase in risk compensation, the concept described in Chapter 4 that applies to people engaging in higher-risk activities when related aspects of those activities are made safer—such as using a condom while having sex with a casual partner, or driving faster when wearing a seat belt. An official from the European Commission explained how, "in the gay community, prevention just went out the window as soon as the drugs came in: now you could have sex without condoms again, and, 'Yee-hah!' That's why it's so dangerous. HIV/AIDS needs prevention in spite of the drugs."[7] The problem may be further exacerbated by the fact that, "as HIV-infected people on antiretroviral therapy become healthier, they are likely to become more sexually active, potentially creating additional opportunities for HIV transmission to occur" (Gayle and Lange, 2004:6).[8]

A way around this for the ART advocates was to promote treatment and prevention within the context of each other. An infectious disease doctor explained the philosophy: "What I am sure of, maybe because I've been working at primary care level, is that no matter how well you do your prevention effort, people will only generally speaking bind to that if there is some hope of proper treatment. Prevention and cure, prevention and care, go hand in hand. But with HIV, we had a lot of care, pastoral care, faith-based organizations and so on; but there was no treatment, so there was no hope. And I think that if you're 15 years old, you're not thinking about if I get infected I'll get care, but somehow collectively in the population the fact that there is care, accessible care, affordable care that will be sustained, perhaps that may influence some change, some prevention. Let's say the message around prevention will become more legitimate if there is a strong message about care. I think that's why we need both."

In a similar vein, a policy advisor for Oxfam saw the current interest in ART as a unique moment in the history of AIDS that must be seized, not just for prevention and treatment but also as part of an even wider package:

> I think that at the moment we've got a fantastic opportunity, and my concern is that let's hold it now before crying for it when it goes. You know, let's hold it now and make it work now. This opportunity is not going to happen again. This is one opportunity; we have never had anything like that on health. Never, ever. So let's grab that opportunity and make it work. Not just for treatment, but for the whole dealing with HIV, for the orphans, for prevention, for everything else. For people to die in dignity. For people to have some food who are HIV-positive. For a whole comprehensive package. So what I am saying is that, let's grab the opportunity and use it.

A spectrum of thinking existed, therefore, from those who argued for prevention in spite of the drugs, to those who suggested that treatment legitimized prevention activities, to those who argued for taking the opportunity brought about by the increased funding to create a comprehensive package for tackling all aspects of AIDS. Advocates for scale-up contended that weighing prevention against treatment was a "sterile debate" based around a "false dichotomy" (Garnett, 2003). And as the debate evolved, this view—that prevention and treatment are intimately linked to each other, and that, in the age of ART, you cannot have one without the other—became increasingly established.

(ii) The risk of generating drug-resistant virus

The very rapid rate of HIV replication imposes great demands on patients taking ART. If they are to avoid the development of drug-resistant virus, such patients must take at least 95 percent of their medication on time, every day, for the rest of their life (Paterson et al., 2000). Otherwise they face not only the prospect of treatment failure, characterized by multiple OIs and eventually death, but also the possibility of transmitting drug-resistant virus to other people, rendering them, too, unresponsive to treatment (Laing and Hodgkin, 2006). Thus, ART programs must ensure both that health systems function effectively so as to ensure a continual supply of drugs, in perpetuity, and also that everything is done to help individual patients to take their drugs as prescribed, for life. Furthermore, national ART policies must be established in order to counter the danger of unregulated drug provision, which has been recognized as a risk factor for the development of resistant virus (Harries et al., 2001).

Evidence focusing on individual-level experiences (as opposed to health-system issues) was used by advocates such as Mark Wainberg in Ottawa to argue that adherence levels would be high in Africa. In the words of a Professor of International Health, "[T]here's increasing evidence in the literature that actually African-based patients are better compliers than Europeans and Americans who are taking ARVs. There are anecdotes that are getting quite wide coverage now of people who sick up their tablets, and they just wash them and swallow them down again, because they are so motivated to keep HIV at bay."

This issue was nonetheless a major concern for a number of my respondents. A Professor of Communicable Diseases was concerned not about individual-level adherence but about the state of the larger health system. "There was an article in *The Lancet* this week," he told me, "saying Africans are very good at taking their treatment. Well, I'm sure they are, when they're made available. But how are you going to logistically do that in a health service that can't provide anti-malarials?" In this regard, the inherent weakness of Uganda's health system was well illustrated in late 2004, when the national referral hospital at Mulago completely ran out of oxygen supplies for patients undergoing surgery (*Monitor,* 2004). If such basic provisions as antimalarials and oxygen cannot reliably be made available, the argument ran, what hope could there be for ensuring supplies of some of the world's most sophisticated pharmaceuticals, along with all their associated paraphernalia?

The worries were not only felt by Western scientists. A London-based Ugandan explained how, "I was one of the people when it started who was quietly advocating for no treatment in Africa. My feeling then was that we cannot afford it. The people would get a pill here and a pill there, and then we would start getting the problems of resistance, which is exactly what is going on now. And then we start fighting a different virus altogether, which you cannot afford to do. So I was one of those who was saying please don't take treatment to Africa. Because we won't be able to control it. But anyway, it's one of those things that you quietly thought about, but you couldn't say it."

Suboptimal adherence is potentially the Achilles' heel of the entire global ART program. As explained above, ARV-resistant virus can emerge even in highly controlled treatment environments (Weidle et al., 2002:38), a fact that only fuels the fears of people like the doctor in Masaka who told me in 2004 that, "in five years, I think we'll probably be worse off than we are now." In fact, her gloomy prediction has not come to pass: widespread, clinically significant resistance to ART has not (yet) emerged in the country. Nonetheless, the threat remains real, and as long as ARVs are in circulation—which, it seems certain, will be for a very long time—constant vigilance will be required to ensure that this inherent programmatic vulnerability does not negate their effectiveness.

(iii) Doubts over ART program sustainability

Finances may have become available from 2002, through the Global Fund and PEPFAR to support a large scale-up of ART throughout Africa, and further cuts in the price of generic ARVs were brought about by a successful legal campaign against two major pharmaceutical producers, mounted by South Africa's Treatment Action Campaign (*Guardian,* 2003), but the promises of financial support to procure these cheaper drugs were not open-ended. The Global Fund itself relies on continuous fund-raising efforts, and PEPFAR was initially guaranteed to run for only five years, until 2008.[9] While the moves toward equitable provision were therefore progressing very well, serious questions were being raised about the extent to which this would be sustainable over the longer term. And, ironically, the problem of sustainability would be exacerbated by the very success of the program, as people who once would have died would now live. Consequently, the numbers of people in need of treatment would grow endlessly as new patients continued to come "on line" while the old ones lived on. An article in the *Lancet* put it succinctly: "Unless annual HIV incidence falls sharply from its current level of five million, treatment programmes will be unable to keep pace with the number of people in need, and will become financially unsustainable" (Gayle and Lange, 2004:6).

A European Commission official cautioned that longer-term thinking is required in order to avoid the serious social and medical consequences that would inevitably arise if funds are not continually forthcoming for decades ahead. "It will grow until it's unsustainable," he explained. "People will say 'this is costing too much, we already have X,000 people on treatment, the economy cannot support this anymore.' And then you're going to have to start saying no to people: 'Sorry, we can't treat you, somebody has to die before you can get treated.' And that's an interesting scenario that people will have to think about. But how to protect against that is to ask how much can you afford in 20 years time. Don't put people on treatment today that you can't afford to have on treatment in 20 years time. Everybody has to think like that."

This very practical, financial mentality was of course not shared by those in the humanitarian camp, for whom equitability should be the aim at all costs, and for whom a belief that things would somehow work themselves out in the future was the basis for urgent action today. In the words of a delegate at a WHO conference on ART operational research (OR) that I attended in Kampala in December 2004, "we need to think about sustainability but that shouldn't make us not act. You have to just start because you don't have an alternative—it's an emergency. Don't worry about funding at this stage, because the funds will be forthcoming. We need to put the fire out now, not worry about whether there will be another fire tomorrow."

Almost nobody was arguing that ART should be withheld from Africa altogether; rather, the issue at stake was the speed at which scale-up should take place. The cautious scientists called for the greatest care and deliberation now in order to avoid more serious problems further down the road, while the humanitarian activists called for urgent action now, and for an improvised, ad hoc approach to dealing with whatever unknowable problems might arise in the future. In the event, the humanitarian view won out, the dice are cast, and any longer-term difficulties that may arise will simply have to be faced.

Unfortunately, it seems we may already have encountered a return to chronic funding shortfalls for AIDS control activities in Africa, thanks to the global financial crisis that began in 2008. A report from Médecins Sans Frontières (MSF), published in November 2009, highlights the increasingly precarious pecuniary situations circulating around major donors such as the Global Fund and PEPFAR (MSF, 2009). PEPFAR, for example—Uganda's principle supporter for treatment scale-up—has now decided that it is necessary to "flat-fund" (i.e., not to increase funds to) its programs in the country until at least 2011. The implications for Uganda are already being felt. Some ART providers have had to cease enrollment of new patients altogether—which means that these people are likely to die—while others can only take on new patients in the event of "attrition." In other words, someone already receiving treatment must either die or become lost to follow-up (ibid.:12). This is precisely the dire state of affairs foreseen—already in 2003, when I interviewed him—by the European Commission official quoted above.

Few people have known HIV for as long as Wilson Carswell, the Scottish surgeon whose prescience at the start of the Ugandan epidemic foreshadowed much of what subsequently emerged; and he is not optimistic about the future of the epidemic. "My money's on HIV," he told me candidly. "HIV beats WHO any day. It's like Manchester United versus Carlisle. I mean, even if you're from Carlisle, you're not going to bet on them, are you?"

Engines of Change: The Big Men of International Politics and Finance

In the end, '3 by 5' did not achieve its stated aim of having 3 million people on treatment by the end of 2005—there were around 1.3 million people receiving ART by that date (WHO, 2006b). However, '3 by 5' did succeed insofar as it created a political climate in which governments and other health care providers were supported to put as many people on treatment as possible, and through which considerable financial and human resources were mobilized. It also acted as a concrete "step towards the goal of making universal access of HIV/AIDS prevention and treatment accessible for all who need them as a human right" (ibid.). Why and how did this happen?

Humanitarian imperative played a central role in establishing a global discourse around the issue, and the fall in prices along with the demonstrated feasibility of small-scale provision served to bring this imperative clearly into the light of day. But nothing would have happened from there had not two factors come together: international political will and funding. Politics and finance tend to be the domain of what could be described as "Big Men"—powerful men at the summit of their respective, highly influential professions.[10] Muraskin (1996) details how such individuals from the pharmaceutical industry and various UN and funding agencies worked—sometimes in harmony and sometimes in conflict—throughout the 1980s to develop the Children's Vaccine Initiative (CVI). This was a more technical process than ART scale-up has been, in that it involved the funding and development of heat-resistant vaccines that would not require a cold chain. With the equivalent technical issues already resolved with ART—triple therapy had been in use since 1996—the debates around providing the drugs in developing countries were both far more public and far more political. Nonetheless, a similar principle applies to ART as it did to the CVI: Big Men decided that the time had come to take action, and action was therefore taken.

Two examples of such Big Men are given here to illustrate how powerful men overrode the ART doubters, imposed their will, and effectively became the engines of change for global scale-up. It should be stressed that there is no intention in any way to denigrate either of these two men through what is presented. This applies especially to WHO Director General Lee Jong-wook, who died suddenly in May 2006. The purpose of including these examples is simply to illustrate how powerful men can work to bring about the things that they want to see done.

As suggested above, an international political framework was provided by '3 by 5.' The rhetoric around the initiative was intended to act as an inspiration and to offer leadership, with WHO's Dr. Lee stating that, "to deliver antiretroviral treatment to the millions who need it, we must change the way we think and change the way we act"; and UNAIDS Executive Director Peter Piot adding that this was "a massive challenge, but one we cannot afford to miss" (WHO/UNAIDS, 2003:1). However, many people were highly skeptical about whether '3 by 5' was a viable target. A co-organizer of a conference I attended in Florence in January 2004, on securing treatment and care for people living with HIV in low-income countries, asked how many of the 100 delegates present at one session thought that the '3 by 5' target would actually be met; only two people put up their hands. This had nothing to do with the scientific reasons given above—people simply did not believe that it was logistically feasible.

Discussions at WHO headquarters in Geneva in February and April 2004 suggested that many insiders felt similarly. One respondent explained that when Dr. Lee was interviewed for the job of WHO Director General, he had not even mentioned '3 by 5' or ARVs as a priority issue; but once in the job, he had been persuaded by his close advisors to take it up as a major concern of his administration. The public rationale was, my respondent said, that "this is a disease that needs serious attention, and we must address it—whether we succeed or whether we fail. And if we fail, we shame the world."

However, there were also internal reasons for pushing WHO to take on '3 by 5,' he said, since it "could serve to unite people within WHO" around an important humanitarian initiative. That said, there was nonetheless considerable resistance within the organization, partly for the scientific and programmatic reasons given in the section above, but also because of something much more mundane: funding. "The mechanisms in the Global Fund aren't in place yet," my respondent explained, "and there's not enough flexible money in WHO. A couple of hundred million dollars, if spent right, could really get this started well, but it's not available, and the result is that people in WHO see '3 by 5' as a threat, since it may cut into their funding. Therefore it has in fact divided people in the organization. It's a question of robbing Peter to pay Paul."

Such was the lack of support for the project that, as another staff member explained, a two-day retreat had been organized for all WHO personnel involved in '3 by 5.' There Dr. Lee had addressed his staff, telling them in no uncertain terms that "if you don't believe in '3 by 5,' you don't belong in this organization." He was effectively forcing his will onto his workforce, and apparently creating some resentment in the process. One female employee spoke with exasperation of working with such "alpha males," while another was more forthright, describing Lee as a "dictator." At the time of my interviews in Geneva, WHO staff were being dispatched to countries all across the globe to provide technical assistance to Ministries of Health as they completed their applications to the Global Fund. "I spent this morning," one respondent told me, "going to various people and asking if they're free and willing to travel next week—not that they have a choice, because if the DG[11] says it, you have to do it and drop everything else."

Even if '3 by 5' was seen as flawed by many people, and even though it created some internal friction within WHO, the political framework it provided did create a unified global target. As such, it worked together with the developments in the financial framework that were already underway to create the momentum that led to global scale-up. The key move in the financial sphere, as explained above, was the decision by Cipla pharmaceutical company to produce cheap generic drugs. This stimulated an enormous increase in the money that was made available by donors: cheaper drugs are very attractive from a donor's point of view, since they provide more patients treated for their dollar. As the Oxfam policy advisor explained, "look at what happened when the prices came down. Three or four years ago, I remember the time when we were talking about ARVs, and people were saying—I mean, even us here in Oxfam—'My God! How do I talk about ARVs?' People just scream and say that these people have no food, have no sanitation, no water, what the hell are you talking about? But now it has changed. And I think Dr. Hamied in India[12] has made history, by his cutting down the price, jumping from $10,000 to $300 [per patient per year]. That just made everyone say, 'ah, right, okay, we can't say no now, we have to think about it.' That really made a big difference."

One of the people who made the call for increased funding for ARVs on the basis of these cut-price generic drugs was economist Jeffrey Sachs. Formerly Special Advisor to UN Secretary General Kofi Annan, he has an extensive track record of advising economies in crisis; and one respondent explained how he had participated in the process of scaling up ART. "You can influence them [the donors]," she told me, "by knowing which part of academia is listened to; and you know that economists are gods, that's how it is. It was only when Jeffrey Sachs came into it—I mean, you like Jeffrey Sachs or you don't like him, my God, his ego is beyond any belief!—but what he did, which is excellent, is he got these [economic] figures on the agenda." Sachs' work in this regard included the first systematic calculation and projection of the money that would likely be needed by 2007 and 2015 for HIV prevention, care (e.g., of OIs), and treatment with ART (Sachs, 2001:163).

A colleague of Professor Sachs in New York explained how he works. "For Jeff, [scaling up ART] is all about money. He's aware of all the complexities, but he doesn't have a lot of patience for them. For him, it's basically just about getting the donors to cough up. And the thing that makes our life a bit complicated now is that he's enormously pro '3 by 5.' I think that's partly because of his personality, his temperament, because this is something that he can push for. It *is* about money, it *is* about getting something done, it *is* top down—which, by the way, is what Jeff likes—and it doesn't get you sucked into some complicated vortex of human behavior." In essence, therefore, Sachs did the sums, put the numbers on the table, and pushed—hard and loud—for someone to provide the cash.

Dr. Lee and Professor Sachs were just two of a number of other financial and political Big Men who forcefully imposed their will and overrode the doubts of their colleagues and subordinates. Muraskin (1996) describes how the Children's Vaccine Initiative was "a tale of strong-willed individuals who worked within the confines of larger social, economic and political structures but who, nevertheless, 'made history' by their actions" (ibid.:1718). A similar phenomenon was observed here; but to Muraskin's observation it could be added that the Big Men who brought about ART scale-up were in that rare position of being able actually to change the social, economic, and political structures that determined what would be done. In other words, rather than having agency merely to act within the structures of their professional world, they had agency to change those very structures, thereby creating an entirely new framework within which they and everyone else would subsequently be obliged to act.

What Was the Role of Research?

The main engines for global ART scale-up were therefore political and financial. Given this, to what extent did research also play a role? It could be argued that the broad failure of efforts to demonstrate the effectiveness of HIV prevention interventions (as discussed in Chapter 4) created an environment that permitted ART to come to the fore. ART provides visible results, a satisfying alternative to the ongoing and rather exhausting uncertainty about HIV prevention. "Failures do not matter," a public health doctor in London explained. "Failures, we drop. We don't ask why did that fail, what can we learn from that? But with treatment, we see people improving. We don't need a randomized controlled trial. You just give them the tablets." In this sense, therefore, research played a role in ART scale-up not through what it did, but what it had *not* done—or, perhaps even, *could* not do.

These limits inherent in some of the more traditional approaches to AIDS research have by now been quite widely recognized, and consequently there has been a shift in the type of work being conducted by many groups. For example, through its fundamental orientation toward improving programmatic approaches and processes, Operational Research (OR)—defined as "the science of better" by the Institute for Operations Research and the Management Sciences (INFORMS, 2004)—has become increasingly relevant for large-scale ART provision. A WHO background document explains that "operational research is a central element in the 'learning by doing' approach to scaling up treatment and prevention. This notion recognizes that incomplete evidence should not constrain scale-up, provided that efforts are made to actively monitor what is happening in countries, learn from comparisons of different programs and policies, and inform decisions" (WHO, 2006c).

The Drug Access Initiative discussed above, for example, made some critical points—based on OR-approaches—which, according to an official from the Uganda AIDS Commission, were "very helpful" in terms of defining ART policy in the country. This groundbreaking project established the fact that ART could feasibly be provided in developing countries, and the major scientific paper that emerged from it positively assessed patients' responses and survival rates (Weidle et al., 2002). Nonetheless, the work was conducted under highly controlled conditions, and serious problems were identified over and above the encouraging headline results—most worryingly, high levels of drug resistance among project participants. As such, it did not provide a blueprint for the way global scale-up should be conducted.

Perhaps more influential in terms of global advocacy was a study describing a successful ART project run by Médecins Sans Frontières in Khayelitsha township near Cape Town, South Africa. ARVs were first prescribed there in May 2001, a step that was "motivated by both humanitarian and public health principles," but also with the objective explicitly "to demonstrate that the use of antiretroviral therapy at primary health care level was feasible, affordable and replicable" (Kasper et al., 2003:20). In other words, this was a project conducted for the purposes of advocacy, and to that end, operational data were collected in order to demonstrate a point that MSF wanted to make. Data from the first 180 patients to be placed on treatment in Khayelitsha were published, demonstrating a significant increase in CD4 cell counts[13] alongside concomitant falls in the rate of OIs such as TB, and also death. The main conclusion of the paper was that "antiretroviral therapy can be safely and effectively used in resource-poor settings, and the time has come to scale-up from pilot projects to widespread access" (ibid.:21). This point was taken up as a rallying cry for MSF and other ARV advocates. In the words of Ellen 't Hoen, formerly Director of MSF's Paris-based Access to Essential Medicines campaign, "[T]hese people are doing very well. A very important message is to show that the drugs can be very effective even in very poor settings" (Guardian, 2002).

I put this to a Professor of Communicable Diseases who had previously told me of his skepticism toward ART scale-up. Surely the Khayelitsha study proves that it can be done? "Yeah, 180 patients," he replied. "But what's the good of that? That's all very well, but when they scale that up to a couple of million people . . . The trouble is, if you say these things, if you voice any of these concerns, you're immediately accused of being a racist, or that you're saying Africans are stupid and all this. So it's difficult to say. And especially in this atmosphere when it's not science, it's politics that's driving the agenda. This is the trouble; the science has gone out of the window."

Politics was therefore driving the agenda for programmatic work on the ground, and this in turn was driving the agenda for research. It is perhaps inevitable that a major paradigm shift such as that associated with

ART brings about changes both in the practice of health care but also, quite fundamentally, in the way research is conducted. Operational ART research in Africa during the 1990s and very early 2000s was largely carried out by activists seeking to prove an advocacy point: that ART provision was feasible. With that point established, and with ART consequently and increasingly part of the treatment landscape, it then became hard to conduct any sort of research on AIDS without taking ART into account. Thus a form of reciprocity was established between the research and its topic: OR contributed to ART scale-up by showing that it was feasible, which in turn fundamentally changed the face of AIDS research.

Scale-Up in Uganda

While the arguments over the possible risks and benefits of ART scale-up raged at the international level, the first tranche of Global Fund money—$36 million—arrived in Uganda in mid-2003 (Global Fund, 2003), and the in-country process rapidly got underway. As AIDS Control Program (ACP) Manager Dr. Elizabeth Madraa explained, "ministers were not always in favor of buying these expensive drugs. But with this Global Fund cash alongside a further $3 million we got from the World Bank, it looks like we now have the money to do it if we plan carefully" (*New Vision*, 2003a). The Ministry of Health subsequently announced that it intended to place 60,000 people on ART by the end of 2005, as the country's contribution to '3 by 5.'

Meanwhile, in June 2003, the government published its ART policy (MoH, 2003a). It had been produced quickly, before national rollout even began, a fact that stands in stark contrast to the very slow progress made with the country's HIV prevention policy, as described in Chapter 4. The document had been the product of input from a number of actors, including the Ministry of Health, donors, and those groups who were already engaged in provision.

The policy's core values revolved around "equity and universal access" (ibid.:7–8). The money and the means had become available, and the government would simply have to trust that it would continue—even if it was well understood that neither of the two major donors, PEPFAR and the Global Fund, had made any guarantee of providing long-term funding. In this, the new policy implicitly recognized the need for extensive donor support—the country's overall health care funding was estimated at just $13 per year for all diseases, of which $8 was provided by the patients themselves, and $5 by the government (ibid.:5). Thus, even with the enormous reductions in price of ARVs noted above, they were still completely out of the reach of most of the 100,000 or so Ugandans who needed them. Provision would have to be free to the provider if true equity was to be established, and this would be expensive: a comprehensive service includes not just the drugs, but also counseling, testing, clinical diagnoses, prophylaxis and treatment for OIs, food supplementation, and community-based alternatives to institutional care and support.

A phased rollout was planned, starting with the regional referral hospitals, then moving out to the district referral hospitals, and subsequently down to Health Centre IV level—simple sub-district clinics run by medical assistants. Peter Mugyenyi—who, in addition to running JCRC, was also Chairman of the technical committee overseeing ARV rollout in Uganda—explained at the Uganda Medical Association's annual conference in Kampala in December 2004 how improvisation and creativity were sometimes necessary in order to expand treatment opportunities for patients. He gave an example of how a British research group had wanted to conduct an ARV study at JCRC with 1,000 new patients, and had complained to him that there was insufficient space at the facility. That was correct at the time, Mugyenyi agreed, but he asked the visitors to return the following week: "Then we'll have space," he told them. And indeed, when they came back, JCRC had raised a large tent in the grounds, big enough to deal with 1,000 outpatients. The research group acceded, the study started, and another 1,000 Ugandans started on ART. "We must not be setting up sub-standard services," he told the meeting, "but I don't allow infrastructure to be a constraint" (Mugyenyi, 2004).

Figure 5.1 shows the rate at which Uganda's scale-up process actually took place—thanks to such creative approaches—and it demonstrates remarkably steady progress toward the policy target of equity and universal access. This was both because the drugs were increasingly available throughout the country, and because they were being provided free to an ever-increasing number of people.

Uganda became one of a small handful of countries not only to meet but to exceed its '3 by 5' target: instead of the expected 60,000 patients on ART, 67,000 Ugandans were registered as ARV patients by December 2005. According to Dr. Elizabeth Namagala, senior medical officer for the ACP, "it was easy to increase the number of patients on ART once we managed to get sufficient support" (East African, 2005). Indeed, one Ugandan doctor explained to me that with so much money suddenly coming into the country, "now it's a question of too much money. Everyone is wanting to fund us. For the first time I was in a place where they were fighting, not for the money, but for the patients."

However, while these figures are extremely impressive, the rapid scale-up of ART stretched an already overburdened health service yet further, and placed

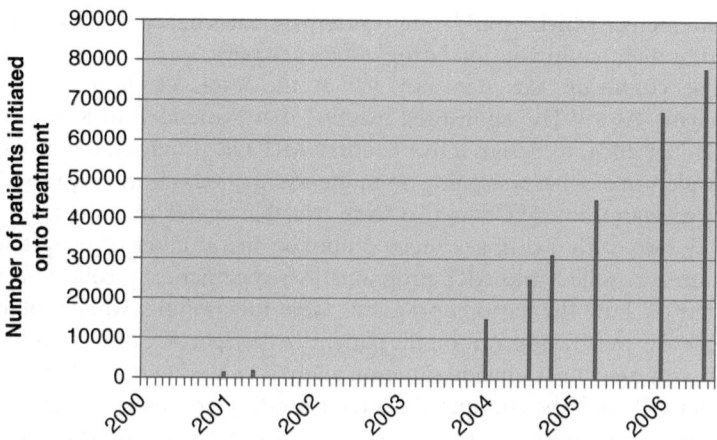

Figure 5.1   ART scale-up in Uganda, 2000–2006.

Sources: Whyte et al. (2003); IPPPH (2003); Uganda Medical Association annual conference (December 2004); East African (2005); and Monitor (2006).

enormous pressure on medical staff. One doctor in Kampala equated the increase in patient numbers at her facility to a "silent tsunami"; and the word "overwhelmed" was being heard with ever-increasing frequency in relation to ART provision in Uganda. This had implications for the long-term sustainability of the program, not least because as AIDS-related mortality rates fell, ever-increasing numbers of patients would require ART. And if medical staff were to find themselves struggling to provide all these patients with adequate adherence support, the possible development of drug-resistant viral strains would be greatly increased.

Another problem was that the rapid scale-up of ART provision was accomplished at least in part by giving providers a great deal of freedom in determining how best to provide the drugs to their patients. Many different modes of delivery and care therefore evolved, with each major provider[14] following different operating procedures. Some provided the drugs and laboratory services for free while others charged; some used generic drugs while others used only the more expensive branded drugs; some worked only out of the clinic while others provided community outreach. And, just to complicate matters further, some providing centers worked with two or more different funding organizations. This means both that doctors in the same clinic might work under different bureaucratic requirements, and also that two people living under the same roof could be attending the same clinic on the same days, but taking completely different ARV regimens. These could have different timing and nutritional requirements, which would only exacerbate the challenge they already faced in maintaining optimal drug-adherence rates.

The confusion was not only felt at the levels of individuals and clinicians. At a WHO-sponsored meeting that I attended in Kampala in December 2004, to design a five-country ART OR program, the lack of a clear picture of what was going on in the country was clearly expressed by the Ugandan team. The data that were available tended to come from the supply side, with a primary focus simply on the number of people who had been enrolled into ART programs. No systematically collected data existed on how the various programs were functioning, what problems the medics were facing, nor on the patients' experiences. Consequently, the team proposed a nationwide situation analysis as a prerequisite before any further OR could be conducted. As their funding proposal explained, "no systematic attempt has yet been made to document exactly who is doing what and how, and consequently the Ministry of Health does not have the information required in order to plan and execute a fully sustainable and effective ART program for the country" (MoH, 2005:7).

In other words, just months into the country's national rollout program, not even the ACP authorities themselves had a clear picture of what was going on. Developments on the ground had far outstripped the central knowledge base, and research was now required in order to ensure that the national ART policy target of equity and universal access could be achieved and maintained over the long term. History was, in a sense, repeating itself: just as HIV prevention activities had been conducted on a wide scale for many years without any clear evidence of effectiveness—as detailed in Chapter 4—ART rollout had been instigated on the basis of an urgent need to act rather than on a firm foundation of evidence. Furthermore, even at that stage there was no comprehensive national plan for monitoring and evaluation.

This was the inevitable result of Uganda's rapid scale-up, but, as JCRC director Peter Mugyenyi explained, it had been necessary for humanitarian principles to take precedence over everything else: "Action had to be taken expeditiously as in all emergencies that cost human lives, irrespective of some possible errors. In such a disastrous situation it is more important to act quickly than to perfect the science and have lengthy plans to avoid any inadvertent mistakes. A scientifically meticulous response is not always possible or desirable in cases of emergency!"

Uganda Cares—The Birth of an ART Provider

The final section of this chapter brings us back to the local level in Masaka, and to a case study of an innovative ART provider that not only promised equity but also guaranteed sustainability: Uganda Cares. The birth of

Uganda Cares illustrates how processes similar to those described at the international level with regard to '3 by 5' also took place at the national and local levels. The story at its essence involved a humanitarian drive that was facilitated by powerful political and financial backing, that faced resistance from a variety of actors, and that finally emerged through the determined work of a diverse group of highly driven individuals.

Many paths—from international, national, and local levels—came together to bring Uganda Cares to Masaka. Internationally, the primary actors were associated with the Los Angeles-based AIDS Healthcare Foundation (AHF), the largest single provider of AIDS care and support in the United States, with expenditure in 2004 amounting to $92 million (AHF, 2005). Inspired by the 2000 International AIDS Conference in Durban, AHF Director Michael Weinstein and his colleague Henry Chang established a subsidiary organization called Global Immunity, based in Amsterdam, with the objective of providing free ART in the developing world. With a long and varied history of AIDS work behind him—including stints in Dr. David Ho's first HIV lab, in Los Angeles,[15] community-based activities in the U.S. gay community, and later with Dupont pharmaceuticals in Uganda and Nigeria—Chang was asked to take on the role of Global Immunity's Executive Director. He already knew some of the important actors in Uganda's health services from his time with Dupont, and was familiar with the country's success in combating AIDS, as well as its openness to foreign assistance. His personal experience of Uganda therefore put the country at the top of the list of possible sites for Global Immunity to start work. How then did Uganda Cares come to Masaka, the site of Global Immunity's very first clinic?

The connection to Masaka came through the Chairman of the district, Vincent Ssempijja. In 2001, Ssempijja had been invited to speak about the impact of AIDS in Masaka at a conference in Los Angeles, where a chain of meetings led him by chance to the President of AHF, Michael Weinstein, whose offices were nearby.

"Michael gave me a full day," Ssempijja told me, "first with some staff, and later on just the two of us, and he wanted to know what was going on in this country. He had some brief knowledge of Uganda—he knew about the President, how he had come out to talk about AIDS, and even to tell the whole world that his country was facing a whole problem when other countries were denying. All the political leadership to the grassroots, from top to bottom, it was an agreed policy that we must inform our people and in fact tell the whole world. That is how I came into contact with Michael." Ssempijja's visit to Los Angeles was fortuitous for both sides, since it provided AHF with a powerful local-level individual who could facilitate the fulfillment of their vision in Uganda, and it provided

Ssempijja with the priceless political prize of bringing the country's first free ART provision to his district.

With this starting point, a meeting on HIV/AIDS Care and Support was co-organized[16] by AHF and Global Immunity in Entebbe in September 2001, attended by 300 participants from 20 countries. As well as bringing together interested parties from all over the region, Global Immunity announced their intention to provide 10,000 Ugandans with ART, specifically the poorest of the poor, those who would not otherwise be able to access the drugs. The organization was to be called Uganda Cares, a name inspired by that year's World AIDS Day slogan: "I care. Do you?"

One of the major innovations of Uganda Cares was a promise to fund treatment not just for the few years of a funding cycle but for life, thereby becoming the very first group in Uganda, perhaps in Africa, to seek to guarantee both equitable and sustainable treatment. Henry Chang explained at the conference that the first Uganda Cares center would be opened in the grounds of Masaka Hospital in less than three months, on World AIDS Day, 1 December. "Our concern is that very many people are dying because they cannot access HIV/AIDS drugs," he explained. "We should strive to provide life-saving mechanisms now and the Ministry of Health and my organization will soon finalize the financial details of this joint venture" (*New Vision*, 2001).

This, therefore, was the public proclamation, which suggested that the deal was effectively done, and that come 1 December, Uganda Cares would open the doors to its clinic in Masaka. However, a great deal of negotiation—including overcoming some considerable opposition to the idea—still remained to be done. President Museveni had opened the Entebbe conference, and Weinstein and Chang took the opportunity to arrange to meet with him the next day to discuss their program proposal. But when they arrived at State House, Henry Chang told me that "we were surprised to see that there were a number of other groups also present." These other groups included WHO, UNAIDS, and USAID, as well as senior officials from the Ministry of Health. The President was "very enthusiastic" about AHF's proposal to start a free ARV program, Chang explained, and it was clear that Museveni felt this was a sufficiently important issue to require representation and discussion between all the central stakeholders. As a senior Ministry official who was also present explained, "the President's view was that the government has a policy of partnership, in order to rally support. So he was happy to accept it."

The enthusiasm toward the project was not, however, shared by everyone in the room. In the presence of Museveni, a representative from the Uganda AIDS Commission warned that "even if the President has said this will happen, you mustn't expect automatically that it will." And a UNAIDS official was even more straightforward in her criticism, saying simply that "you will fail in your enterprise." Such doubts were also shared by people who were not at the State House meeting, including an AIDS social scientist who told me that the promise of free ARVs made the fledgling Uganda Cares an "object of derision."

Why was there so much resistance to the idea of providing life-saving drugs to dying people? As a Ministry official explained, "people at programming level—knowing about prices, system requirements, health infrastructures, the need to have laboratory equipment in place—these people said they were too ambitious. So I can understand why they were wary." I put this point to a Uganda AIDS Commission executive, and asked if the skepticism was due to worries about the likely success of the project. "No," he replied. "It was simply a question of losing power."

Thus the resistance among the major actors—both Ugandan and international—appeared to be derived both from a sense that their turf was being invaded, and also from very practical concerns about the viability of such an ambitious project. In relation to the latter, it is undeniable that neither Global Immunity nor AHF had any institutional experience of Africa at all. However, it could equally be argued that it was precisely the unfettered idealism and hope that came with this inexperience that permitted them effectively to break the rules of what could be done, and to overcome the conservatism that was the natural domain of the long-term actors. Weinstein and Chang had an idea, they visited Uganda, met the President, offered their plan, and it was accepted. As Chang explained, "the way we moved into Uganda was a great example of how political will can make something happen. Global Immunity circumvented the standard protocol for changing policy, and went straight to the President."

But even with the promise of substantial and indefinite funding from abroad, with President Museveni's unequivocal national-level political support, and with a District Chairman willing to provide the necessary local infrastructure, Uganda Cares' birth pains were far from over. As one of the medics involved at the start explained to me, "we had a tug of war to start it. Even the Ministry was not supporting us. They said 'the drugs are so expensive, there's no way you can do it free of charge, it's not sustainable.' But we had people who wanted to support us, so we said if we can treat 100 people, why shouldn't we do that? We said we can allocate a building for the work—one of the private wards—and storage space. But the Ministry resisted, and it didn't auger well. It took the intervention of State House before we could get accredited. The Ministry said we didn't have the capacity. So we said, 'who is supposed to provide the capacity? You!' Anyway, we had the people to do the work." He was talking about events in 2001 and 2002, but Ministerial resistance had not entirely diffused even in late

2004. As a Kampala-based public health doctor told me in October of that year, "as things stand now, Uganda Cares hasn't really gone to the core of the Ministry. To Director or Commissioner levels. They think this thing is not feasible, but rather that we have to do it for political reasons."

Nonetheless, the top-level political support from President Museveni forced the issue through, and the Uganda Cares clinic was opened in Masaka by First Lady Janet Museveni in February 2002, just five months after Chang's initial announcement at the Entebbe meeting. As Vincent Ssempijja told me, "Global Immunity is really very fast. We have worked with many, but they were really very fast." Scale-up during the first year was, however, slow, as the team developed their protocols and operating procedures. They were, after all, pioneers in providing free treatment to a general population in Africa, and, furthermore, they were developing a comprehensive ART program before the country even had an approved national ART policy. The first draft of the Antiretroviral Policy for Uganda was not available until June 2003 (MoH, 2003a), with the first edition of the National Antiretroviral Treatment and Care Guidelines for Adults and Children following in August 2003 (MoH, 2003b). In other words, Uganda Cares was effectively operating within a policy vacuum for nearly 18 months. One of the results of this was that some of their earlier patients started with what eventually became the nationally designated second-line treatment. Once the guidelines were published, there was debate among Uganda Cares medical staff about whether or not to downgrade these patients back to the new official first-line treatment. In order to reduce their risk of developing resistant virus, it was decided to keep them on second-line therapy.

After 12 months, 11 Uganda Cares patients had died—mostly because they started treatment too late—but 100 remained on the books, of whom 80 were adults and 20 were children. Clinical improvements had been remarkable, with average CD4 counts increasing from 51 to 310 after one year of treatment, average weight gains of 11.3 kg over six months, and—critically—average patient adherence levels exceeding 95 percent, meaning that that the specter of resistant virus would be held at bay (IPPPH, 2003:30).

Another important aspect of the early period of operations was overcoming resistance from other local service providers. I asked District Chairman Vincent Ssempijja how they had tried to work around the doubts expressed by some of their local peers.

> At that time [he explained], people had already done a lot of work—the donors and the NGOs. But what they were doing was counseling, educating the patients on how to live positively with AIDS, and then also treating the

opportunistic infections, the fevers and the coughs. And also educating the masses, and looking after the sick by giving them some little food. That is what the NGOs were doing, and they had already gone very far. Now somebody comes and says we need to look at treating. It was different to what was happening. So these people looked at it, they were skeptical about it. And others were looking at it and, to be frank, they were not happy. They were envious. They thought maybe it was going to interfere. Despite what they were doing being very good, it was work, it was employment for them. I think you understand what I'm saying. Somebody coming to treat these people with ARVs is going to cause the other processes to become outdated or even stopped. And if you bring somebody who is going to treat people, he is going to get a lot of recognition.

So that was there, and I saw it. I saw it very early, and Weinstein and Chang saw it also, and they suggested we had to use these NGOs who had been doing all this work, and use them on this one. How do you get the patients? Do you just announce on the radio? No, there are already these bodies who have been working with these patients in these other fields. They know them. Why don't we bring them onto a coordination committee, get those patients from them, get those who have already reached that level for treatment, let them recommend them? And we really need to continue with preventive measures, because if you can prevent the deadly disease from entering your body, the better. And we need to continue counseling, and educating the masses how to look after their relatives.

There was a lot of work to be done, but these people had that fear which we really tried to solve by bringing everybody on board, by explaining that these kind of preventive methods are very important, even more than before, so let's work together. So harmony came back, and we used the best method really. We got people without bias, and that is how we succeeded.

Thus, at the local level, an attempt was made to address this resistance by establishing partnerships with the organizations already working in the field. To this end, all Uganda Cares clients were referred by another local service provider, who had previously been providing them with medical, psychological, and/or nutritional support. Since most patients were therefore being served by more than one provider, cooperation between doctors from the different groups was ongoing with regard to individual patients. I observed this while accompanying a palliative care doctor from Kitovu Mobile Care Unit as she travelled around the district, and several times she spoke of the need to check certain details of individual cases with one of the Uganda Cares doctors. Through this regular contact and cooperation, the doubts that I understood from various sources had existed at the start of Uganda Cares operations were dissipated, to the point where the organization has now become an essential component of local AIDS service provision.

With the basic programmatic procedures in place, and the potential clinical success of the project established, Global Immunity increased funding levels so as to facilitate a scaling-up of activities. By July 2004, Uganda Cares in Masaka was treating 802 clients; and the numbers continued to grow toward the estimated 8,000 people in the district who, according to the District Director of Health Services, were in immediate need of treatment.

The work of Uganda Cares has therefore born fruit in Masaka, but it has also spawned free ART centers elsewhere in Uganda as well as further afield, thus meeting one of the organization's stated objectives: "To develop a replicable and scalable model of HIV/AIDS clinical care appropriate to the safe and effective provision of ARVs in resource-constrained settings" (IPPPH, 2003). The Minister of Health, Mike Mukula, called Uganda Cares a "proven initiative" in September 2003 (*New Vision*, 2003b)—irrespective of the continuing doubts of some of his Ministerial staff—and personally participated in organizing for the second Uganda Cares clinic to be opened in his own home district, Soroti, in November of that year. As one of my respondents explained, "Captain Mukula said even my people are suffering, so that is why Soroti was second. In the third world, it depends really on personal input. Because we don't have enough, it depends on who is there first, it depends on who really shows interest and hard work." Six years later, in August 2009, 12 Uganda Cares sites were running throughout the country, providing ART to nearly 16,000 patients (AHF, 2009); and Global Immunity itself was operating in seven other African countries.

A senior Masaka doctor summarized how Uganda Cares had stimulated a change in thinking at the national policy level. "We were the first in the country to give treatment for free, and for the general community. And now, we are there, and WHO has said we are one of the best practices. And I think this is what made the Ministry wake up. This was the start of the movement to provide free ART in the country. If we had agreed with the Ministry, we would not be having free treatment now all over Uganda." This view was endorsed by a public health official in Kampala who said simply, "Uganda Cares played a very big role—they made the Ministry to run!"

Discussion

Analysis of the material presented in this chapter shows that while the scale of events with respect to the evolution of ART policy and practice may have differed between global, national, and local levels, there were a number of striking similarities in the processes at each level. Three areas are discussed in this concluding section in order to demonstrate these similarities, as well as to highlight some of the particular differences between the levels. The three areas are: (i) the importance of key individuals, or Big Men, as engines of change; (ii) research and the use of evidence; and (iii) resistance to ART scale-up and how it was overcome. Through this discussion, the interconnected nature of events, as well as the importance and power of networking within and between levels, is also underscored.

With respect to the first area of similarity, the drive for ART scale-up at each level was driven primarily by the decisions of key individuals in positions of political and financial power. These individuals have been characterized here as Big Men, men in the worlds of politics and finance with both the power and the will to fundamentally change the structures in which they work. As Muraskin (1996) points out, social science often views people as having agency to act within the confines of the social, cultural, and economic structures that they live in, but here it was the other way round. By working within powerful advocacy coalitions (Sabatier, 1993)—groups of like-minded people working toward a common policy goal at each of the three levels—elite groups of Big Men collectively and irreversibly changed those structures.

At the international level, the Big Men included—among many others, and presented here in no particular order—Dr. Hamied, CEO of Cipla pharmaceutical company; Dr. Lee Jong-wook, former Director General of WHO; and financial guru Professor Jeffrey Sachs. These men, as well as the other major players at the international level, would all have known *of* each other, but would not necessarily have known each other personally; and certainly they would not all have met together more than a handful of times to discuss global ART scale-up. In this sense, the international advocacy coalition was looser than those at the national and local levels, where personal and professional ties among many of the major actors have tended to be closer, if for no other reason than geographical proximity. Nonetheless, the objective that the international Big Men collectively worked toward—mass treatment of people living with AIDS in developing countries—was clear and based on what they saw as an unambiguous humanitarian imperative. It was this shared purpose that facilitated their cooperation.

At the national level in Uganda, the Big Men came from the political rather than the financial sphere, since funding for ART programs has tended to be almost entirely donor-driven. Thus Ugandan financiers have not played a significant role. These political actors included President Museveni; Crispus Kiyonga, the former Minister of Health, who facilitated the Drug Access Initiative; and—if politics can be defined as the art of getting people to do what you want them to do—Peter Mugyenyi of the

Joint Clinical Research Centre. In Masaka, the key political actors were local—most notably District Chairman Vincent Ssempijja—although it should not be forgotten that Uganda Cares would never have flourished without strong national-level support, directly from President Museveni. For similar reasons to those given at the national level, the most important financial actors at the local level—Michael Weinstein and Henry Chang of AHF/Global Immunity—came from the international level.

This illustrates the dependency of national and local-level political actors on financial support from the international level. But it should not be forgotten that the international financiers also needed the political support of national and local-level politicians in order for them to meet their own objectives. These may all have been Big Men, capable of changing large social and economic structures, but they were all also people who were dependent on other people. International Big Men need local Big Men to cooperate with them if they are to succeed—and vice versa. Even Big Men cannot operate effectively by themselves. Critically, too, their various breakthrough decisions could not have been made without the supportive ideological context that had been established by the army of activists working in the international AIDS advocacy coalitions.

With respect to the second area of similarity—research and the use of evidence—the first point to note is, perhaps rather obviously, that there would have been no scale-up of ART provision at all if the drugs had not been developed in the first place. ARVs were the product of a major breakthrough in clinical AIDS research, which in this sense was therefore the ultimate prerequisite for any sort of policy or programmatic development at any of the three levels.

The role of research as an actor in the scale-up of ART did not end once the drugs existed and their clinical efficacy had been established. The many people who doubted that large-scale ARV provision was feasible in Africa were countered by a small group of scientists who actively set out to demonstrate that it could be done. To this end, operational studies of small pilot projects—such as the DAI in Uganda (Weidle et al., 2002), the Khayelitsha project in Cape Town (Kasper et al., 2003), and the first year of Uganda Cares operations in Masaka (IPPPH, 2003)—played a critical role in proving the naysayers wrong by demonstrating clinical success among their patients, and thereby providing important evidence for use by advocates and the Big Men.

A four-step process of research can be described, which applies equally at each of the three levels:

1. The researchers involved in the various programs had a pre-existing ideological position that favored large-scale ART provision;

2. They implemented an ART program, partly for the patients in their clinics, but also in order to show to a wider audience that their ideological position was grounded and workable;
3. The clinical successes that they demonstrated justified the arguments of activists, politicians, and financiers who wanted to scale up ART provision;
4. On this basis, political, financial, and logistical support for ART scale-up emerged, facilitating the process to begin.

The evidence was therefore produced with an explicit agenda: it was to be presented as an advocacy tool that would provide the justification for action. As such, it contributed significantly not only to legitimizing the scale-up of ART programs but also to establishing international, national, and local-level ART policies. With the AIDS treatment landscape fundamentally and permanently changed as a result, it also subsequently changed the nature of AIDS research itself.

Having argued that evidence contributed to bringing about ART scale-up at each of the three levels, however, it would be misleading to suggest that the development of large-scale ART programs was evidence-based. The pilot studies noted above focused almost exclusively on clinical outcomes for small-scale provision, and there was no substantive basis for arguing that the successes would necessarily be repeated across the board when tens, or even hundreds of thousands of people were being treated. As with much of the HIV prevention work described in Chapter 4, ART scale-up was conducted primarily out of an urgent need to act, rather than on a firm evidence base. The evidence that was used certainly helped to kick-start scale-up, but it could not, by its very nature, make any definitive claims about the likely success of large-scale provision.

The third area for discussion concerns resistance to ART scale-up, as well as the process of overcoming it. Resistance was faced at each of the three levels, but the reasons for it differed from one level to the next. Internationally, some of the strongest objections were voiced by scientists concerned about the potential public health ramifications of a scale-up process that lacked a stable foundation. By contrast, the worries at the national level in Uganda, and locally in Masaka, tended to be political and practical. Politically, there were turf issues, with some of the groups who already had many years of experience in treating people with AIDS fearing a loss of power, financing, and prestige. Practically, there was unease about program sustainability, the capacity of health systems to deliver on such an ambitious agenda, as well as the possible impact on other important health care concerns if too many of the country's doctors were to move exclusively into ARV provision.

Overcoming the resistance to scale-up—or, in some cases, pushing it through regardless of the resistance encountered—took a different course at each of the levels. Internationally, it is notable that the doubters tended to be non-African public health scientists and clinicians with significant hands-on experience of health care in Africa.[17] In spite of their important knowledge and experience, however, these people are not, as a group, powerful decision makers. Those whose very job it is to make decisions, and who pushed ART scale-up through—the Big Men—had, in stark contrast to the public health scientists, lived their professional lives far away from the day-to-day reality of health care provision in Africa. Regardless of this fact, they imposed their will and overrode the concerns of their worried subordinates. The scientists' long-term public health concerns of what might or might not eventually happen as a result of rapid ART scale-up were far less politically attractive to the Big Men than the tangible and immediate outcome of treating and saving dying patients by the thousand—today.

In Uganda, the government resisted ART scale-up primarily because of concerns over sustainability: What would happen to the tens of thousands of patients who would be receiving treatment if funding suddenly dried up? These worries were effectively made redundant by Peter Mugyenyi's illegal importation of cheap generic drugs into the country. This forced the government into a politically uncomfortable corner, from which they had little choice but to permit the importation of these and subsequent shipments of ARVs, even though this went against the instincts of many senior officials in the Ministry of Health. Mugyenyi's actions demonstrate how the determination of one well-placed individual—either because of, or in spite of breaking the law—can overcome strong resistance and bring about a major policy change at the national level.

Locally in Masaka, the field of play was far smaller, and it was possible for the Uganda Cares leadership to act in a more consultative fashion than was possible at either the national or international levels. Resistance was dissipated by bringing in the other AIDS service providers as collaborating partners in the ART provision process, thereby offering them an active stake in the project, and ensuring that their work and livelihoods were not threatened.

6

The Masaka Intervention Trial: A Case Study in the Interpretation of Complex Research Findings

Introduction

The previous three chapters have presented the life stories of three different AIDS control policies in Uganda and have examined the extent and means by which they have been influenced by research. This chapter looks at the issue from the opposite perspective, by taking an individual research project and examining the extent to which it may or may not have influenced policy. I personally worked on this study in Masaka over a period of five years with a team from the Medical Research Council (MRC) Programme on AIDS in Uganda. It was a community-based project called the Masaka Intervention Trial (MIT), and it evaluated two different approaches to HIV prevention.

I applied to join the MIT because it was asking a critical question in a high-prevalence area—*How can we reduce new HIV infections?*—and because it was using hard, biological indicators within a strong epidemiological methodology that would theoretically be able to provide a definitive answer. I, and many others, believed that the interventions we were evaluating were likely to be effective, that we would be able to demonstrate their effectiveness, and through this that our work would have an impact on HIV prevention policy both in Uganda and further afield.

But it did not work out this way. For a variety of reasons, the MIT results—the product of over a decade of work with the involvement of literally tens of thousands of people—met with little more than a shrug from the Ugandan authorities, and a flicker of international- and local-level interest, followed in turn by silence. This chapter aims to investigate why this was so.

In order to provide the context and rationale for the study, the chapter starts with an introduction to two other community-based trials that evaluated HIV prevention interventions—in Mwanza, Tanzania; and in Rakai, Uganda—since the three studies are often discussed in relation to each other. The MIT's design and implementation are then briefly described, before moving to the reaction, interpretation, and impact of its findings from the perspectives of some of the stakeholders involved. These include scientists, policy makers, and people living in the study communities. In addition to demonstrating the way in which complexity of findings can affect the extent to which a study is taken into account during discussion about policy, the chapter also demonstrates the great diversity in perspectives of a trial that involved the participation of many thousands of people.

"How Can We Reduce New HIV Infections?" The Mwanza, Rakai, and Masaka Trials

As described in Chapter 4, a reasonable amount of African AIDS research had been conducted during the late 1980s and early 1990s, but most of the work was quantitative, descriptive, cross-sectional, and based on convenience sampling methods. No substantive evidence existed at that time regarding the effectiveness of the various HIV prevention strategies that were being used. One of the reasons for this was that it was predominantly scientists from European and U.S.-based research institutions who were defining the research agenda and, with an eye firmly on the need to publish, they were flying in, collecting the most accessible data, and quickly flying out again to conduct their analyses. They had no personal stake in the disaster they were investigating, and as one British scientist who had worked in Uganda at the time told me, they "left little behind but anger and confusion . . . Northern scientists were not always welcome in Uganda."[1]

The gap in pertinent knowledge was underlined by findings from an investigation by WHO's Global Program on AIDS (WHO/GPA), which reported that "of the AIDS research done in sub-Saharan Africa in 1988–89, nearly 95 percent of the 559 projects identified were of no immediate relevance to the local populations" (cited in Southern African Economist, 1992:5). Serious ethical issues were also emerging in African AIDS research. In the words of a Kenyan sociologist, "[W]e have knowledge, but what do we do with it? Doctors take blood and go away; social scientists ask questions and go away. But the community is still dying" (Barnett and Blaikie, 1992:174).

Meanwhile, there were increasingly stark warnings for the future. Jonathan Mann, head of WHO/GPA, warned that "the pandemic not only remains dynamic, volatile and unstable, but it is gaining momentum—and its major impacts, in all countries, are yet to come" (ibid.:176). In February 1992, WHO estimated that 12 million people were then infected worldwide, of whom 7.5 million were Africans. But by the year 2000, they warned, "approximately 25 million African infections could be expected" (Weeks, 1992:208).[2]

The root of the problem was the fact that HIV incidence rates remained extremely high in many parts of Uganda, as well as elsewhere on the continent, in spite of widespread educational efforts and consequently relatively high levels of knowledge about HIV and AIDS. In other words, there appeared to exist no straightforward, linear relationship between high levels of knowledge and safe sexual behavior. Some of the easier research questions had by now been answered—*who is at risk of infection* and *how are they being infected?*—but the ultimate question remained unresolved: *How can we reduce new HIV infections?*

This was the context in which the idea for the MRC's MIT was born. Since 1989, the Kyamulibwa cohort's[3] annual sero-surveys had been providing insights into the dynamics of the AIDS epidemic in this rural area. But as one WHO official told me, "there had been criticism that the MRC had milked the epidemiological side of things without providing much in the way of interventions." The most appropriate next step in the MRC's research strategy was therefore deemed to be an investigation into HIV prevention; and on this basis, the first steps toward conceptualizing and designing a major prevention study were taken in 1992.

The range of available HIV prevention options was very narrow at this time, with behavioral change—specifically delaying sexual debut, limiting numbers of sexual partners, and using condoms—on the one hand, and the prevention and treatment of sexually transmitted diseases (STDs) on the other.[4] The options may have been few, but that did not mean that many rigorous evaluations of these intervention approaches—investigating whether or not they actually worked, or, indeed, if perhaps they may have unexpected and harmful effects—had actually taken place. A handful of studies evaluating the efficacy of condom use among sex workers had been conducted in Africa (Moses et al., 1991; Pickering et al., 1993; Laga et al., 1994; Asamoah-Adu et al., 1994), but nobody had yet attempted to evaluate a wide-ranging behavioral intervention—sometimes referred to as IEC, or Information, Education, and Communication—in a general population anywhere on the continent. Since such interventions were going on regardless, the practice of HIV prevention activities had thus moved "ahead" of research into HIV prevention activities, and it was important to address this discrepancy (Oakley et al., 1995).

With respect to STD prevention and treatment, work had begun in November 1991, on a major trial in Mwanza, Tanzania (see map on page xv), to evaluate the efficacy of syndromic STD management[5] as a means of reducing HIV incidence (Hayes et al., 1995). The syndromic management approach was a concept supported by WHO (WHO, 1991), and it was believed by many public health workers to be well suited to poorly resourced, rural clinics in Africa. The Mwanza trial—explicitly intended to "provide valuable data for health policy makers" (Hayes et al., 1995:919)—was conducted by a collaborative international team, including German, Tanzanian, French, and British researchers from the Tanzanian National Institute for Medical Research and the London School of Hygiene and Tropical Medicine.

The Mwanza trial was underway by the time discussions had started to design the MIT, and, in the words of a WHO official who had been involved at the time, "the MRC wanted to respond to Mwanza." The fact that the MRC Programme on AIDS in Uganda also had strong connections with the London School of Hygiene and Tropical Medicine, as well as with WHO/GPA, greatly facilitated the incorporation of a syndromic STD management component into the nascent MIT:[6] it was believed that two large studies evaluating the same intervention would carry a great deal of weight in the minds of policy makers. As a former senior MRC member of staff explained to me, "the STD trial simply had to happen." The STD intervention was to include training in syndromic management for health workers in health facilities in selected study communities—or parishes[7]—as well as ongoing support and the provision of appropriate antibiotic drugs.

An IEC component was included in the trial on the basis—as explained above—that individual-level sexual behavior change was then the only other major strategy available for HIV prevention, and yet it had never been subjected to a rigorous evaluation in an African population. Its inclusion also meant that the Masaka trial would be more than a mere replicate of the Mwanza trial. As the former MRC official explained, "nobody had an answer for IEC, and nobody else was looking for it. In any case, locally it was very easy to accept the IEC bit, as this was really all that was being done in Uganda at the time in prevention, so it was easy to explain to people. So the timing was right."

With technical and financial support from WHO/GPA, as well as scientific input from colleagues in London, the trial gradually came together. Data from the Kyamulibwa cohort helped establish appropriate treatment algorithms[8] for the various STD syndromes in order to ensure that the right drugs were prescribed; and a WHO consultant with considerable experience of IEC in Zambia flew to Uganda in July 1993, to offer advice on the study's behavioral component. "We wanted to make the community IEC intervention as standardized as a tablet of chloroquine," he told me. The idea, therefore, was that each of the study parishes selected to receive the IEC intervention should have the following:

1. An AIDS Prevention Committee (APC), consisting mainly of parish-level politicians who would meet once every three months, and who would offer local legitimacy to the operation;
2. A Parish Coordinator (PC), a full-time individual who would oversee all study activities and act as the point of first contact for the MRC in his or her parish;
3. A group of around 25 Community Educators who would provide information and advice, mainly on a one-to-one basis, for people living in their community; and
4. A drama group consisting exclusively of local talent, who would be trained by an MRC drama consultant to perform a set of specially written plays in each study village.

These people received a small allowance to maintain their motivation (from roughly $3 every three months for each of the APC members to about $70 per month for the full-time PC), while regular training and support meetings with each group in each parish provided the opportunity for MRC staff to keep in touch with developments on the ground.

Certain other principles were also established for the IEC package, including the recognition that since Ugandan men tend to have more control over sex than women—in terms of whom they have sex with, when, how often, and how—it would be vital to include a high male-to-female "agents of change" ratio if an effective message was to be put across to the community. With this in mind, 16 individual topics were selected by MRC staff with assistance from the WHO consultant, and standardized messages about them were developed for dissemination in the study communities. They included—among others—how HIV is and is not spread, STD treatment-seeking behavior, marital faithfulness and reducing number of sexual partners, abstinence, and condom use (Kinsman et al., 2002:256).

The study design was finalized by the end of 1993. The MIT was to be a three-armed community randomized trial,[9] with each of the three arms to include six noncontiguous parishes. The study's stated aim was "to determine whether IEC programmes alone, or in combination with improved STD management, are an effective intervention against HIV-1 transmission in an adult population where the primary transmission of HIV-1 is through heterosexual contact" (MRC, 1992:19). One of the three study arms

ARM A	ARM B	ARM C (Control group)
6 parishes = about 32,000 people - Behavioural change (IEC) alone	6 parishes = about 32,000 people - Behavioural change (IEC) + syndromic STD management	6 parishes = about 32,000 people - Non-HIV-related community development activities

Figure 6.1   Schematic representation of the Masaka Intervention Trial, showing the interventions conducted in each of the three study arms.

was to receive IEC alone (Arm A); one was to receive the same IEC package but with the addition of syndromic STD management in government and private clinics (Arm B); and the third was to act as a control group, in which non-HIV-related community development activities were to be promoted, such as fish-farming and rabbit-rearing (Arm C) (see Fig. 6.1). For ethical reasons, condom promotion and Voluntary Counseling and Testing (VCT) were instituted in all study arms.

Approximately 32,000 people lived in each of the three study arms. In order to attain sufficient statistical power to measure the impact of the interventions, the direct involvement of around 4,500 adults from each arm would be required. Thus, a total of around 13,500 individuals were to be censused, interviewed, and bled by members of a survey team (which conducted its work entirely independently from the groups conducting the intervention itself) two or three times over a mean follow-up period of about four years.[10] Through this, it would be possible to accurately ascertain HIV and STD incidence and prevalence rates in each arm for comparison, and also to estimate changes over time in reported sexual behavior for every participating individual. Great importance was also placed on an operational research component: "In designing and implementing the study, every effort will be made to ensure that the approaches employed are appropriate and affordable under the present conditions in Uganda, so that the lessons learned from the trial can help improve the quality and scope of IEC and STD interventions elsewhere" (MRC, 1993:2). Full details of the study design are given in Kamali et al. (2002).

Thus the ground was laid for the MIT, but the project took some time to take off. Referring to the trial's slow start, an internal WHO/GPA report from 1994 stated that "it is evident that the need for human resources to manage and implement the interventions had been greatly underestimated when the original budget was prepared." Additional funds were subsequently earmarked,[11] and the team was expanded.

While the MIT was gradually gaining momentum, the Mwanza trial had been concluded, and the results were published in the *Lancet* in

August 1995 (Grosskurth et al., 1995). It was reported that syndromic STD management had reduced HIV incidence by a full 42 percent, a finding of huge significance: "This is the first randomized trial to demonstrate an impact of a preventive intervention on HIV incidence in a general population" (ibid.:530). The accompanying editorial carried the almost euphoric title, "STD control for HIV prevention—it works!" (Laga, 1995), and for the very first time in the African AIDS epidemic, there was a sense that the continually unfolding disaster could perhaps be brought under control. The Mwanza trial results subsequently stimulated a major shift in policy for HIV control in Africa. For example, it contributed directly to a six-fold increase in annual spending on STD control for developing countries by the UK's Department For International Development (DFID) between 1995 and 2000 (Philpott et al., 2002:197).

Back in Masaka, a new MIT Project Leader was installed late in 1995, and although there was awareness that the Mwanza results could have stolen some of Masaka's thunder, work on the trial finally started in earnest. The survey team began systematically working through the study parishes, interviewing and bleeding participants; cadres of health workers were trained in syndromic STD management; and the IEC component was launched. I joined the study in October 1996, initially as a health educator, helping to train and support the community educators, and subsequently as coordinator of the IEC section. We had 560 volunteer workers on the project, of whom, in accordance with our wish for a high male-to-female "agents of change" ratio, 57 percent were men (Kinsman et al., 2002). The MIT also had around 35 paid employees,[12] all of whom—myself excepted—were Ugandan nationals.

With the intervention and its evaluation now fully up and running, a third major trial—the Rakai STD Control for AIDS Prevention Study—was drawing to a close less than an hour's drive down the road. Run by the U.S.-funded Rakai Project, this community randomized trial had also been designed to evaluate the efficacy of an STD intervention as a means of reducing HIV incidence. The intervention strategy here was not syndromic management, however—as in Mwanza and Masaka—but rather mass treatment. This involved administering antibiotic treatment for syphilis, gonorrhea, chancroid, chlamydia, trichomonas, and bacterial vaginosis to everyone in the selected communities, "irrespective of symptoms or laboratory testing" (Wawer et al., 1998:1211). In other words, every adult was to be treated for these STDs, whether or not they had symptoms of disease or were actually infected at all. The rationale for this shotgun approach was to reduce the overall prevalence of treatable STDs in the population—several of which do not always produce symptoms—which, it was hypothesized, could subsequently reduce the incidence of HIV.

The Rakai study had run between December 1994 and mid-1998 and, like the other two studies, was designed explicitly "to provide the scientific basis for policy" (ibid.:1222). When the results emerged, however, the policy implications were not at all obvious. The Rakai trial found that HIV incidence was identical in both the control and intervention arms (Wawer et al., 1999), which, put simply, meant that the HIV prevention intervention had been ineffective. The explanation given by the researchers was that HIV infections in Rakai tended to occur independently of treatable, bacterial STDs. In other words, these did not act as significant cofactors for HIV infection. Thus, reducing their prevalence would have no impact on HIV incidence, a finding that stood in direct contrast to what had been found just along the lakeshore in Mwanza.

Possible reasons for this discrepancy were vigorously examined within the scientific community, with many people concerned that the Rakai results could undermine the global policy interest in STDs that had been generated by Mwanza. One WHO scientist spoke of a meeting he had attended to discuss the Rakai findings, at which the best means of presenting the data had been discussed. "It wasn't an easy meeting," he told me. "We almost had fist fights," because the Rakai Project representatives reportedly wanted to say that STD control "doesn't work . . . The only thing we did manage to do was to get them to change the title of their paper, so it no longer said 'STD control is not effective.'"

Uncertainty over STD treatment as a strategy for HIV control gradually gave way to a satisfactory explanation for the findings, which allowed for both Mwanza and Rakai to stand uncontested. The lead scientists of the two studies coauthored a paper in which they asserted that "the divergent results may be complementary rather than contradictory" (Grosskurth et al., 2000:1981), their conclusion resting on two points. First, the Mwanza trial took place during an earlier phase of the epidemic than the Rakai trial: computer modeling had suggested that the contribution of STDs to HIV transmission decreases with the maturity of an HIV epidemic (Robinson et al., 1997). And second, the prevalence of genital herpes was much higher in Rakai than in Mwanza, a critical point since herpes is a viral disease that is by definition not amenable to antibiotic treatment, and so was not targeted in either Mwanza or Rakai. Genital herpes is also implicated as a major cofactor for HIV infection (Fleming and Wasserheit, 1999). These two points combined to demonstrate the importance of epidemiological context as a determinant of the likely effectiveness of an STD-oriented HIV prevention intervention. This was a crucial intellectual breakthrough, leading away from the rather simplistic one-size-fits-all approach that had prevailed after the Mwanza findings were published.

In this sense, some international public health experts saw that significant positive spin-offs had evolved out of the Rakai controversy. "I remember shaking when Rakai came out," an English epidemiologist with long experience in Mwanza recalled. "The fear at that point was that, look, if ever there was proof of a disarticulation between STDs and HIV, this is the proof. But the sky didn't fall in, because there was a really plausible explanation for it. What it did was it made people to lift up their eyes from the specific STD-HIV interaction, and focus more on the context. And then people started to talk in terms of the age of the epidemic. And now there's this whole discussion about phase-specific intervention strategies."

The American scientist who was acknowledged by the Rakai team as the one "without whom we never would have realized this study was possible" (Wawer et al., 1998:1223) agreed. "The emerging consensus prompted by those trials showed how thinking had matured," he told me. "Surprise, surprise: it's not simple!"

The Masaka Intervention Trial—Findings

The whole Mwanza/Rakai debate took place in a world far distant from Masaka, where, in June 2000, the scaling down of the MIT survey and intervention activities began. But we, as MRC, were well aware nonetheless that the scientific environment into which our results were to be placed was quite different from the one in which the study had been designed back in the early 1990s, in large part because of the Mwanza and Rakai trials. And although the controversy between the researchers involved in those two studies had been resolved, some people still saw the STD-HIV debate in Africa as stalled, with the score at one "for" STD control (Mwanza) and one "against" (Rakai)—notwithstanding the fact that these were two different interventions in two epidemiologically distinct populations. The MIT—with a Mwanza-type intervention in a Rakai-type population—was to be the decider in relation to STD control as a means of reducing HIV. Thus there were high expectations for the trial's STD results.

There also seemed to be interest from some quarters with respect to the MIT's IEC component. Referring to our intervention, Harvard-based researcher Ted Green wrote, "I suspect that this traditional or culturally tailored interpersonal approach has had significant impact. Research-based evaluations will probably be able to prove (or disprove) this hypothesis" (Green, 2003b:174).

And so, with the final survey in the final study community complete, the substantial task of analysis began. We were confident that both the STD and the IEC interventions had been satisfactorily implemented. Process data collected throughout the trial showed that 12,200 cases of symptomatic disease had been treated in the six STD communities—as compared to 11,600 cases in the Mwanza trial (Grosskurth et al., 1995:532); while in the twelve IEC communities, we had recorded 81,000 IEC activities, with a total of 390,000 attendances. We had also distributed 164,000 information leaflets (Kamali et al., 2002).

The dataset to evaluate the interventions' impact was enormous and complex, including information from over 20,000 people.[13] I asked the statistician who was responsible for the analysis to tell me how she had felt when she finally pushed the button on her computer and became the first person to learn the results of the MIT.

"I was disappointed," she told me. "I think I was expecting a little bit of an effect in terms of reducing HIV incidence, but there was nothing whatever. So, yes, I was disappointed. I suppose I thought that these interventions would have some effect on some people in terms of changing their behavior. Not huge, but some. I wouldn't have been surprised if there was a reduction in HIV incidence, but it hadn't been [statistically] significant. But in Masaka there was no reduction at all."

I very well recall the moment when I too found out the results some time later, in the company of the MRC's Programme Director and the MIT Project Leader. Leafing through reams of computer printouts, I searched item by item and mostly in vain for the magical signature of success: "$p<0.05$," the indicator of what is conventionally held to be a statistically significant difference between variables. Key among the points of interest to us were the differences in HIV incidence rates between Arms A, B, and C, but no such statistical differences were to be found, meaning simply that the interventions had not had the desired effect. There were some signs of success buried in other areas of the dataset, as explained below, but some of these were, at first sight, counterintuitive, and they only complicated the interpretation further. At the end of our meeting, the Programme Director put the printouts—still under embargo—carefully back into his brief case, the Project Leader gazed silently out of the window, and I left the room thinking of all those many years of hard work by so many people and how it seemed to have come to nothing.

The view of the WHO consultant who had assisted with the study design nearly a decade earlier was that "the Masaka results were all over the place." It would be hard to argue with this assessment, with the study's main findings summarized as follows (see also Table 6.1):

1. There was no difference in HIV incidence between the three study arms. Since HIV incidence was the study's primary outcome measure, this result was enormously disappointing in purely human terms,

Table 6.1   Incidence Rate Ratios[a] for HIV and other STDs between Study Arms of the Masaka Intervention Trial

	Arm A vs. Arm C	p-value[b]	Arm B vs. Arm C	p-value
HIV incidence	0.94	0.72	1.00	0.98
Genital Herpes incidence	0.65	**0.003***	1.00	0.99
Active syphilis incidence	1.02	0.92	0.52	**0.044***
Gonorrhea prevalence	0.64	0.26	0.25	**0.013***

[a] The incidence rate ratios (IRR) in this table offer a means of comparing the incidence rates for particular diseases in Arms A and B (where the interventions were conducted) with the incidence rates for the same diseases in Arm C (the control arm, where no intervention was conducted). An IRR of less than 1 in this case indicates a protective intervention effect, while an IRR of more than 1 points to a harmful intervention effect. In either case, the p-value has to be less than 0.05 if the effect is to be seen as statistically significant.

[b] Statistical convention holds that there is a *significant* difference between two variables only if the p-value is less than 0.05 (marked in the Table in **bold** and with a *).
Source: Adapted from Kamali et al., 2003.

as we had not managed to avert any new HIV infections within the study population itself. But it was also politically very challenging, since at face value it suggested that the Ugandan model for HIV prevention—which was broadly what we had been evaluating—did not work in an experimental setting. If that was indeed the case, what were the implications for Uganda's position as the African AIDS success story? And what would this mean for the many other African countries that were seeking to emulate the Ugandan model? A satisfactory resolution was achieved, however, by putting the findings into the context of data collected from the Kyamulibwa cohort. The Kyamulibwa data—collected in an area of Masaka district far removed from any MIT activities, and therefore "uncontaminated" by the interventions—had shown a significant decline in HIV incidence throughout the period in which the trial had run (Mbulaiteye et al., 2002). This naturally falling incidence was very likely also to be taking place in our study parishes, and we concluded that the interventions we had implemented in Arms A and B were simply insufficient to reduce incidence yet further (Kamali et al., 2003).

2. A reduction of genital herpes incidence was shown in Arm A (the IEC-only intervention arm), but not in Arm B (the IEC + STD intervention arm). We could reasonably have expected to identify a reduced level of new genital herpes infections in *both* Arms A and B, due to the broader sexual health messages we were putting out in these two study arms. And had we shown a reduction of genital herpes only in Arm B, this could plausibly have been explained as a

cofactor effect in relation to the successful syndromic management of the other (bacterial) STDs. But we were unable to offer any convincing explanation for the anomalous reduction of genital herpes incidence in Arm A only.

3. The incidence of active syphilis and the prevalence of gonorrhea had been reduced in Arm B but not in Arm A. This, at least, conformed to expectations, since the antibiotic treatment given out in Arm B had specifically targeted these diseases.

Adequately interpreting and explaining all these findings was extremely difficult. Dr. Jimmy Whitworth, the MRC's Programme Director, summarized for me why he believed we had not obtained the positive result that we had all hoped for:

I think that there are a number of things that went on that in retrospect were problems. One of them was that there was a fall of HIV incidence and prevalence across the board happening anyway. And there were reported huge changes in sexual behavior over time. Now I don't believe slavishly all the reports of improved sexual behavior—I think that they're exaggerated by a desirability bias—but I think that they are a marker that there was safer sexual behavior going on already. So in a way, the trial was acting on a slanted table. It wasn't a level playing field. Things were getting better regardless of the trial, so that made it hard to get a result.

The other thing that I think in retrospect is that with regard to the intervention as it was developed, there weren't that many people who were at risk in the population. The intervention was very much a classic ABC,[14] wasn't it? It was delay sex, reduce your number of partners, reduce casual partners, and use condoms; and I think many people—the majority of people—didn't have scope actually to change their behavior. And so there was only a minority of people in that community for whom that message was actually going to make a practical difference. It might have reinforced them to continue, but it wouldn't have made any difference to their actual behavior because it couldn't. So potentially you could argue there was a mismatch between the intervention and the population. The intervention might have been more useful in a population that hadn't already had behavior change, while an intervention that would be effective in the Masaka population would be different.

Presentations of the findings and their interpretation were made to the Ugandan Ministry of Health, at WHO in Geneva, and at the London School of Hygiene and Tropical Medicine; and a paper was published in the *Lancet* (Kamali et al., 2003). Jimmy Whitworth summarized the message that was put forward:

"The essential message to policy makers in Uganda was 'don't change anything, because you're already doing the right things.' What this trial did was that it demonstrated that intensifying those same interventions doesn't add anything further, but keep on doing what you're doing. Please don't throw the baby out with the bathwater. Please don't stop. I think they were pretty positive about that kind of message."

With this, the MIT—whose implementation had cost $1.44 million[15] (Terris-Prestholt et al., 2006:S113)—and the formal dissemination of its findings were concluded.[16]

The Masaka Intervention Trial—Responses and Interpretations

The second half of this chapter will explore the way these results were received by the many stakeholders in the study, and will demonstrate the extent to which different perspectives can stimulate very different responses and interpretations of the same thing.

An important methodological point to bear in mind here is that the enormous range of respondents—from high-profile international epidemiologists in Geneva to poor, subsistence farmers in rural Masaka—made it impractical to ask the same questions of everyone. The overall thrust of my questioning, however, was to elucidate people's perceptions of the trial, and, broadly speaking, to establish what message they had carried from it. At the national and international levels, I was also interested in ascertaining the extent to which the study might have influenced HIV prevention policy.

International level

Most of my respondents at the international level saw the results from the MIT as appearing on a historical continuum: the frame of reference was Mwanza and Rakai, and it was against the results of these studies that they placed the MIT. Probably as a result of these associations, the first mental connection made by many people when Masaka is mentioned is the STD component of the trial: the comment of a Zambian scientist I met at a conference—"Masaka? That was the STD trial, wasn't it?"—characterizes the response of many people. This was significant, since it meant that the IEC intervention—which was considerably larger than the STD intervention, as well as being the very first of its type to be conducted in Africa—was relegated to the back seat.

The first public international discussion of the MIT results took place at the Fourteenth World AIDS Conference in Barcelona, in July 2002, with one full session devoted to attempting to resolve the "seemingly discrepant results of the results of the Mwanza, Rakai, and Masaka STD intervention studies in Africa" (Abdool Karim et al., 2002). Working through the data from the three studies, delegates arrived at a "basic consensus" about the respective results[17] and concluded that "the take-home message is that STD management is both an important component of primary health care in and of itself, and an effective HIV prevention strategy. Its impact will be most prominent in populations with a high incidence of bacterial STIs and a high incidence of HIV" (Rutherford, 2002:85). The point here, therefore, was not to let the Masaka results undermine the principal importance of preventing and treating STDs or, as the MRC's Programme Director had said to me, not to throw the baby out with the bath water.

The MIT findings were subsequently published in the *Lancet* in February 2003 (Kamali et al., 2003), with an accompanying editorial commentary which concluded that, "many people will be disappointed by the lack of reduction in HIV incidence despite an apparently appropriate intervention that reduced other STDs and was implemented on a huge scale with great care and commitment in a stricken country. Perhaps this was the right trial done at the wrong time—i.e. when HIV incidence had fallen well below the expected level, when the contribution of other STDs to continuing HIV transmission had diminished, and when substantial reductions in risk behaviour were already taking place across all communities" (Stephenson and Cowan, 2003:633).

This epidemiologically derived explanation—which broadly concurred with the Barcelona consensus—was strikingly different from the one that was published in an editorial in the *Times* of London that same week. This suggested that the "authoritative" Masaka findings "appear to show that there is no connection between improving sexual safety and reducing HIV rates." The results, argued the newspaper, were "hugely politically sensitive. [African] states which have been unwilling to fight AIDS in the aggressive way the West would like might easily see in them justification for dropping AIDS prevention programmes altogether" (*Times*, 2003a). This message—charging African countries with not following Western-driven AIDS policy directives—was broadened into a more global point by a subsequent letter to the *Lancet*. The author worried that "policy makers might conclude that STD activities should be downplayed . . . If some of the hard-won advances in STD/HIV-1 prevention and control are not to be lost, convincing explanations are needed to account for these findings" (O'Farrell, 2003:2085).

An alternative perspective of the MIT emerged from the ranks of the AIDS dissidents—a disparate group of individuals who believe, among other things, that HIV is not the cause of AIDS (Duesberg, 1997), and that the primary mode of HIV transmission in Africa is not heterosexual intercourse but rather the use of unsterilized needles (Gisselquist et al.,

2003). Speaking to the *Times* on the week of publication of the MIT results, David Gisselquist announced that "results from the Masaka study add to the already long list of findings from other studies that don't fit the hypothesis that most HIV in African adults is from sexual transmission" (*Times*, 2003b). A subsequent paper by one of his colleagues referred to the MIT findings, as well as those from the Rakai trial, as support for their hypothesis: "The HIV theory predicted that HIV was sexually transmitted and therefore AIDS would spread throughout the heterosexual population. This has not occurred. In fact data from the largest, longest, best designed and executed studies available conducted in the USA and Africa show that HIV is not heterosexually transmitted" (Papadopulos-Eleopulos et al., 2004:598).[18] It should be made clear here that no explanation is given as to precisely *how* the MIT results could support such a conclusion, but it was striking nonetheless that it should be given credence in a prestigious, high profile newspaper such as the *Times*.

A critical voice was raised in a letter to the *Lancet* by Powles and Day (2003), who questioned the value of conducting large intervention trials such as the MIT in the first place. They argued that the MRC team had followed an "interventionist view, in which the public only enjoy the fruits of science when they are ministered directly by the intrusive activities of professionals." They compared the MRC's purportedly intrusive approach with "an alternative, less technocratic view, which values the advance of science no less, but which seeks to realize its benefits by creative engagements with all relevant forms of social organization, and not just by professionally controlled interventions. Unfortunately, those who value science seem often to distrust democracy, and vice versa" (ibid.:2086).

I discussed this challenging perspective with one of the authors of the *Lancet* editorial. "He's basically criticizing the people like us who want to do trials," she told me. "You know, 'we're in charge.' And he was saying, 'look, it's not your domain: just give people information, and it will seep into the communities as it clearly did in Masaka, and people will behave accordingly. It's not your right to impose an intervention trial on them.' That was the critical message I got from it, which is fine if you take that sort of leap of faith. But I think you can't do that, as you've got to show that these things aren't harmful." This position represents an important reversal of the initial rationale for the trial, which, as stated above, was "to determine whether IEC programmes alone, or in combination with improved STD management, are an effective intervention against HIV-1 transmission." (MRC, 1992:19). Now, with the results in mind, it had instead become a tool for demonstrating a lack of harm.

While much of the debate in the literature took place in the immediate aftermath of publication, discussion about the MIT within the context of Mwanza and Rakai continued for a couple of years. Most of the published papers on this discussion have been based on computer modeling, and have concerned themselves with STD management as a means of preventing HIV, with a strong focus on maintaining political and medical interest in this approach (White et al., 2004; Korenromp et al., 2005; Hogan and Salomon, 2005; Phair et al., 2005). One article stands out in its determination not to forget IEC, or behavior change, since this "provides a clearer basis than clinical interests such as STD treatment on which to build HIV prevention strategies in Uganda and elsewhere" (Low-Beer, 2004:361).

Turning now from the literature to the views of my international-level respondents, the most positive view of the trial results undoubtedly came from a Ugandan WHO official who had once worked on the study. "It's not a disappointing result," she insisted. "It's a good result. I have no doubt that preventing STDs reduces HIV. And I have no doubt that changing behavior reduces HIV."

A UK-based epidemiologist also drew a very positive conclusion, both in relation to the IEC and STD interventions, and also with respect to the growth of knowledge about HIV prevention in general. "I think what's important is not the message that sexual health promotion doesn't work. Your results and Rakai did not actually translate directly into 'it doesn't work.' You can't equate the two. It doesn't translate into 'we shouldn't do it.' It actually translates into 'yes, but we need more.' It's not a clear message, but in the same way that the maturity of the epidemic came out of Rakai [as an important point], something similar will come out of Masaka. That's no bad thing. The point is that it's all incremental, you just get more data. This to me is like a real-life example of how incrementally you get a better and better sense of approaching reality, approaching what's true, and focusing on issues. I just think that the next trial or big bit of information clears the picture a bit."

A Professor at the London School of Hygiene and Tropical Medicine concurred, adding that we have reached a new level in both our understanding of and our approach to HIV prevention activities. "I think you can say that we've probably gone about as far as we can with this generation of interventions. We need now 'second generation' interventions that are more tailored, and whether that means better STD management, whether it is highly efficacious behavior interventions of some form, whether it's microbicides, vaccines, circumcision, ARVs; this is stuff that all needs exploring. But also I think it's important not to write off behavioral interventions. We've done one behavioral trial, in one population. Now, you wouldn't do a trial using some anti-hypertensive for heart failure, find that it didn't work, and then say that we can write off drug therapy.

Because there are other things you can do, other things you can try, and it's the same with behavioral interventions."

These broadly positive views were countered by the rather less-sanguine thoughts of a senior UNAIDS policy maker. "I'm sure everyone who walked out of the London [results dissemination] meeting came back with a different take on it, and different actionable steps," he explained. "The problem is that something like the Masaka trial didn't have a clear result, and it would be of virtually no value to policy makers, because it could be interpreted in several ways, and it's all so cloudy. I think my biggest take on this is that in the absence of clear findings, everybody will walk away from this with what they want . . . Where you have an absence of a clear, single finding, people will go off and make selective use of data."

According to a scientist working with a U.S.-based AIDS research group, this difficulty of attaining a clear, single finding is largely methodological, and is primarily the result of conducting trials with relatively short-term follow-up. "You need time for it. I think it's bullshit to expect results so fast. I know there's all the pressure, but it's a little foolish to expect results with biological markers in such a short time. It's not worked with any other behavioral intervention. In fact most of the other ones that have worked—like seat belts or not smoking—have been the result of combined efforts over many, many years. Convincing groups of professionals, convincing policy makers, legislation, public education: eventually all of that comes together. People still smoke and people still don't put their seat belt on. But by and large, we've moved in the right direction. I think it is stupid, it is so short sighted, to expect that with AIDS we can do anything faster."

Perhaps the clearest summary point that emerges at the international level of analysis is a picture of people using the MIT findings to support their own pre-established positions. As the UNAIDS executive put it, "in the absence of clear findings, everybody will walk away from this with what they want."

First, there was the epidemiological establishment—led by scientists from the London School of Hygiene and Tropical Medicine—who took the data, along with that from Mwanza and Rakai, to argue for what they already believed to be important: sustaining the focus on STD prevention and treatment. Then came the AIDS dissidents, who argued that the MIT's failure to reduce HIV incidence supported their hypothesis that HIV in Africa is not predominantly sexually transmitted. Next came the anti-interventionist view of the *Lancet* correspondent, who railed about scientists who oppose democracy; and finally, there was the Ugandan WHO official, who stuck to the well-established position regarding the route by which her country has become known as an AIDS success story.

These international-level groups and individuals expressed strongly held opinions, and—rightly or wrongly—the MIT was used in each case as an opportunity to justify and confirm these.

National level

Discussions with actors at the national level were held primarily with policy makers in the Ministry of Health, as well as a few Kampala- or Entebbe-based scientists. I also spoke to a well-respected health journalist who writes nationally, and whose response to my questions about the MIT set the tone for many of the other respondents. Given that there had been a series of dissemination workshops for interested parties in the capital in late 2002, I asked if he knew about the MIT, and if so, how had he interpreted the results? "The details of that one are not clear to me," he answered. "Was it in Rakai or Masaka?"

This sort of answer was echoed by an Assistant Commissioner at the Ministry of Health, who told me he had attended one of the dissemination sessions in Entebbe, but admitted frankly that, "I don't remember exactly what was the result." The point was underlined further by one very well-connected individual in the field, who told me that he thought there are "not more than three people in the Ministry of Health who know about how the Masaka Trial ended."

If that is indeed the case, I interviewed all of the Ugandan policy makers who knew the results; and of these three people, two were highly critical of at least the IEC component of the project. The first one I spoke to followed a line very similar to that of the U.S.-based researcher quoted above, echoing the frustration over a methodology that was almost destined to show failure. "Was four years [for follow-up] long enough? To mould someone's behavior, in only four years? I think that's unreasonable."

This individual seemed not to be especially impressed by the need for research in principle, suggesting that the process was externally driven, with little local, Ugandan input. "Donors have an uncontrolled appetite for research," he said, "and with the research, we become unrealistic about what will work. Still, the Masaka trial was not a wasted effort. There wasn't much," he concluded, "but I wouldn't have expected much anyway."

The second critical voice from the Ministry also raised questions about research, suggesting that the trial had been unnecessary in the first place. "I am kind of familiar with the Masaka trial," he told me when I asked for his reaction to the findings. "But we had a problem with it, as we already know that IEC works. For all health programs, it's obvious that first you must have right knowledge about risk factors and preventive methods."

The third voice of Ministerial officialdom had no direct critique of the trial itself, and although this person suggested that the results have had no impact at all on the practice of STD management in Uganda, he said they have had a marginal impact on at least the rhetoric of policy. We were discussing STD management in Uganda, and the fact that the Ministry of Health policy still adheres to the syndromic approach in spite of the fact that the MIT—the only trial to evaluate this strategy in the country—had shown that it had no effect on HIV incidence, as well as a very mixed impact on STDs themselves. "There was a dissemination workshop in Kampala to which the Ministry was invited," he said, "but has that evidence been put to use? No, there was no subsequent change in focus. We still have to control STDs, to improve general reproductive health, even if doing this is not going to have an impact on HIV. So it is essentially business as usual, although the rationale has now changed." In other words, syndromic management remains an important strategy for STD control in Uganda, just as before; but it is now conducted solely for STD treatment, and not with any suggestion that it may also contribute to HIV prevention.

From the Ministry perspective, therefore, it would seem that the MIT was not in fact a useful tool for anything at all: very little was apparently learned from it, and scarcely anything has changed as a result of it in terms of either policy or practice.

Outside the Ministry, in the world of the scientists, the MIT inevitably stimulated interest among the Rakai STD trial investigators. "In order to understand my impression [of the MIT results]," one of these explained to me, "you must understand the political-scientific environment. The Mwanza results were out, and we had released the Rakai findings at the AIDS conference in Geneva [in 1998], and there was tension between the syndromic management people versus those who supported mass treatment. Therefore there was interest and confusion as to how to interpret our [Rakai] findings. So when the Masaka trial came out, our initial feeling was that now we would be believed, that the Rakai trial results had been confirmed. But equally, of course, we were also disappointed."

By contrast, a mid-level Rakai Project social scientist's relative lack of knowledge about the MIT reminded me of what I had often sensed during my five years in Masaka. She was unsure about the Masaka STD control strategy, and knew little of the IEC work, which highlighted the fact that even though the MRC and the Rakai Project are geographical and methodological neighbors, there was remarkably little crossover of ideas or discussion outside the top echelons of the two groups. Consequently, the teams implementing the work in the field had only limited awareness of what the other research group was doing, and had little opportunity to learn from each other. A short, one-hour drive may have separated us, but a number of people based in Kampala, Entebbe, Baltimore, London, and Geneva were far better informed about the collective nature of the work than were many of the people actually doing it.

Three main points emerge from this brief discussion of the national-level response to the MIT results:

1. There was a relative lack of knowledge about the results among some key individuals, even though the MRC had held a series of dissemination workshops in Kampala and Entebbe. This lack of knowledge extended through several spheres, including otherwise very well-informed people in the Ministry of Health, the media, and other scientists.
2. Some policy makers were actively critical of the principles standing behind the IEC component of the study, arguing that (i) behavior change is a long-term issue that cannot be realistically implemented and then measured during a mere four-year follow-up period, and (ii) that "we already knew that IEC works."
3. HIV prevention policy has not changed at all in Uganda as a result of the study, though it contributed to a shift in the *rationale* for conducting syndromic STD management—its official purpose changed from HIV prevention to wider reproductive health promotion. In that sense, the request to policy makers by the MRC's senior manager not to throw the baby out with the bathwater—"Keep on doing what you're doing, please don't stop"—was heeded.

Local level

My respondents on this topic at the local level can be split into two categories: (i) district-level health and education officials, as well as medics; and (ii) people who lived in the study communities and who worked on the project.

I interviewed seven individuals in the first of these categories (medics and district officials in Masaka) and found very limited awareness about the MIT: only one of the seven knew anything of the study's results. Referring to "this research that was done about whether health education was beneficial," he said that, "for our staff, it kind of put them off. You came out and found no impact." A second person reported good relations and communications with the MRC, and was aware of the Programme's current work preparing for HIV vaccine trials and evaluating the efficacy of vaginal microbicides, but he conceded that he did not know what the MIT had found. "I have those documents," he said, "but I've not had time to go through them in detail. I've not had any discussion about the results." A third district-level official was completely unaware of the MIT. "I have not come across that one," he told me. "But now that you have informed me, I will put them [MRC] to task about it." This lack of awareness at district level is especially striking given that Masaka district was the site of the first and only community-based trial to evaluate an IEC intervention anywhere on the African continent.

By contrast, my selection criteria for interviewing people at village level ensured that they were well aware of the study. The 26 people from this category whom I interviewed—who came from 5 of the 12 study parishes—had all worked on the trial in some capacity, and I used their perspectives partly in their own right, but also as a lens through which to learn how the wider community had perceived the MIT and its outcome.

The first thing I wanted to investigate during my interviews with the former volunteer workers was how the sero-survey process had been understood and experienced by people living in the study areas, since this would provide important context for the way in which people subsequently understood and interpreted the trial's results. As explained above, the survey took place over three rounds, and it involved following up individuals over time in order to determine HIV incidence in the three study arms, and thereby to ascertain the efficacy of the IEC and STD interventions. Extensive community mobilization took place prior to each survey round, and participants in the survey were given compensation for their contribution. This took the form of free access to their HIV test results and related counseling; simple drugs provided by the survey team to treat common illnesses that were prevalent in the community; as well as washing basins and soap.

In some cases, the survey had apparently been seen as a relatively straightforward and uncontroversial process. "It was three exercises [rounds of bleeding]," a former AIDS Prevention Committee (APC) member explained. "At first the community would resist, so mobilization went on. The second round, they came out. But the third round, since they were [by now] fully sensitized, they gave up their blood, knowing that finding out the percentage of the disease in the area [required] first that they gave their blood, so that we can find out the percentage with the virus."

"There was no problem," another former APC member agreed. "People liked to be bled, to know exactly about their blood, whether HIV is within the blood or not. It was good, for that person who is willing to know his status."

There were, however, several instances, and in several study parishes, where there was considerable suspicion about the survey. "There are two different groups in society," a third former APC member told me. "One group realized that research was important, but another bigger group remained thinking that this was not only [for] research. There must be something else connected with money. The small group realized the aim, but then the bigger group felt something was behind it."

This issue of money appeared independently and prominently in a number of interviews. "It was rough somehow," a former Community Educator explained. "People were not willing to listen. Some of those negative people were bitter with the blood samples, they were not happy with it, thinking MRC was taking their blood somewhere to sell it. Some went to an extent of even hiding from the survey team. There were forms where the person who was tested had to sign, and they refused to sign. Some people got bitter, thinking that we [volunteer workers] were conniving with MRC people, and we were given money secretly for each sample. So it became a problem."

Some people in the community found it very hard to understand why such efforts were being made to find and bleed particular individuals: "For us [people who worked as guides for the survey teams], we were getting a little money,[19] so it was OK; and there were also these people from the MRC office,[20] and people saw them and said, 'they are looking very nice and big and fat!' So for us we were uplifted [by the allowances]. But people in our villages can see those differences, and that made it very difficult. They thought that the blood was precious, according to the way they [MRC staff] live, and the amount of salary they get from abroad. And that amount of money makes them to look so well! Whereas, down here. [Shakes head]. So now the common man feels that he is the project of the higher people. The common man here *feeds* the higher people. That is why they struggle, why they drive a vehicle to go to one person who has refused to give blood. Second time, third time, fourth time! They ask why?! Spending all this money on these nice big Land Cruisers and fuel, coming to this person. Maybe there is something!"

The compensation that was offered to study participants—voluntary counseling and testing for HIV, treatment of simple diseases, and washing basins—was in most cases very welcome, but some viewed the package with a degree of cynicism: "There's another incentive which attracted people again. Those were the drugs which the survey team was moving with. Most of our people have got simple sickness, and those simple sicknesses were being treated. So people became eager, and they liked it. In other words, it was another trap!"

These views account for some of the uncertainty felt in the study communities toward the survey, but there were also incidents where people opposed the process more actively—even with threats of violence. "There was one case," a former guide for the survey team explained, "and he was a Moslem. The bleeder[21] went alone, and he told me that the man was about to cut him—he came with a *panga*![22] And the bleeder had to run away! Very near us, up there. He didn't want to be bled."

It should be stressed that these cases represent a minority, and that, broadly speaking, the process was acceptable to the population, with 71 percent, 72 percent, and 91 percent of the eligible participants providing blood samples in Rounds One, Two, and Three respectively (Kamali et al., 2003:648). As a former Parish Coordinator said, "most people still gave us their blood. If you come and talk with a simple tongue, these people will eventually get convinced."

With this high level of participation in mind, I felt it necessary also to investigate the issue of informed consent. Obtaining informed consent is a standard practice in all medical research, and it requires that people agree to take part in a study only if they are properly and fully informed about what it entails, what the possible benefits could be, as well as the risks. On the assumption that the understanding of those people who had worked on the study would probably be better—and would certainly not be worse—than that of the actual study population, I asked former volunteer workers what they thought the trial had been investigating, and why they thought it had been necessary for us to bleed people. People mentioned cure and medicines for AIDS, but not a single respondent said anything about prevention.

As a former APC member said, "after giving [study participants] their results and whatnot, you also benefit from getting your research. And you can get the cure. For us, we don't know about HIV virus, but you people, you are ahead of us in knowing how the virus is, so you can make your research and maybe have the cure. After your research you can get some medicine which cures, and then we can forget all about AIDS!"

A former Community Educator suggested, "[T]hey were looking for the blood to find the people with HIV, so we know what to do with the people who are infected. To make research about whether they can get medicine."

Similarly, a former PC believed that "they wanted the blood because that's where the virus is. To see how many people are infected; and to see whether they can get a medicine."

Clearly, therefore, there were some difficulties both with the bleeding of participants in the study for the survey, and in terms of participants' understanding of what the study was actually about. Nonetheless, there also appeared to be a strong belief among the former Community Educators (as implementers of the IEC intervention) that their work had been useful and valuable.

"The messages we gave were better [than those on the radio]," a former Community Educator told me, "because most people, when they put on such programs talking about diseases, most of them don't listen. They want music. But we went to the people direct. So this type of education did a very big work. We went person-to-person."

Several respondents also appeared to believe that the work had been effective. "As a behavioral change creator," a former member of one of the drama troupes reported, "I have changed people, especially on the side of prevention, using the condom. And for those who are not yet married, all those who are preparing for marriage to go for blood checking. And people have responded, there is a change . . . They are no longer going to the witch doctors for consultations."

I asked this same individual if the MIT's IEC work had contributed to reducing the rate of HIV infections. "Very, very much!" he replied. "People learned so much! When you use drama, you get a certain message. People are so much interested in those drama shows. Now the people of the area know what AIDS is. And they know the way it is spread."

Thus, there seems to have been a disconnection in people's minds between the survey (which people appeared to see in relation to medicine and a cure) and the interventions (which they knew concerned HIV prevention). In fact the two were intimately related, with one measuring the impact of the other. This raises questions about the extent to which people gave truly informed consent when agreeing to be interviewed and bled for the survey. But it may also reflect people's wishful thinking, since the perceived value of prevention is not always as high in people's minds as the perceived value of cure. This point is given a broader context by the work of Linda Stone, who wrote about a primary health care program in Nepal that emphasized disease prevention and health promotion. "All the village health workers I have ever interviewed," she explained, "reported that people are frequently disappointed when they find that the worker will not be performing curative services" (Stone, 1986:297).

My final set of questions to the former volunteers concerned their perception of the study's results. When these had emerged from the computer, and it was discovered that the interventions had not been effective, a series of discussions was held in the MRC Masaka offices concerning how we should provide feedback to the study communities—something we had always promised we would do. The results were, as has been made clear above, epidemiologically complex, and it was concluded that, with all due respect to the villagers who had participated, it would simply not be feasible to explain the headline results of the study unambiguously at community meetings.[23] Instead, we decided to delve into the records for each study village in order to show how HIV prevalence had changed there over the previous few years. We knew that prevalence had decreased over the course of the trial in all the three study arms, so we also knew that such an approach would provide good news to those who had given us so much support through their participation over the years.

However, when asking people about the feedback they had received—albeit three years after the village presentations—it emerged that not all of our volunteer staff actually knew the results. One former Community Educator said he knew "nothing at all" about what we had found; another said she remembered MRC staff coming to give feedback in her village, but "I don't remember details of that presentation."

There were other cases where people did not believe that the prevalence figures we had presented could be accurate. "They said 90 percent of the people were OK," a former drama player told me, "and ten percent were found with HIV." I asked if people had been surprised with that figure. "Exactly!" he laughed. "They were denying it! Just like that! The officials from MRC came to tell them, but they were surprised. They said no, no, no! It should be more than that!" I then asked why people had thought this. "Because of the rate of death, you know. Seeing the rate at which people die."

In another village, with a similar prevalence rate, people also found it hard to believe the results, but for a different reason. "What they told people in our area was that after they bled them, they found that ten percent were infected," a former APC member explained. "But the people did not understand that thing; they said no, it can't be. They said it must be like 60 percent. Because they know their behavior!"

There were, however, also cases where the results were understood and believed, and where people were satisfied with what had been found. "In our parish we were lucky," a former Community Educator told me. "People with AIDS were very few, and K [MRC staff member] told them that the virus is not on a very high speed here. The percentage was fair. This STD treatment, it helped so much. So he told the people to be serious, and not to involve themselves in sexual plays."

The MIT's results may have been complex, and they may have shown that the interventions had had no impact on HIV incidence, but it would be wrong to suggest that there was no longer-term impact of our work at the local level. At least two of the parish drama groups survived and, as of my fieldwork in 2004, continued to perform without any external support, providing a small income for a handful of people. In the words of a policy maker I spoke to in Kampala, "the Masaka trial may have had an effect, just not the one you were trying to measure, or the one that you had expected."

Discussion

The MIT was a large study, using a widely accepted methodology, and asking an important question—*How can we reduce new HIV infections?*—in a heavily affected African country. Two widely adopted and complementary

HIV prevention intervention approaches were rigorously evaluated—Information, Education and Communication (IEC) for behavior change, and syndromic STD management—but the study's finding that these had no impact on HIV incidence brought about no subsequent change in HIV prevention policy or practice. Why was this?

The reason at the local level in Masaka was very straightforward. In spite of the MIT being conducted within the district's jurisdiction, there was extremely limited awareness of the study among relevant district officials. This lack of awareness is particularly striking given that Masaka district was the site of the first and only community-based trial to evaluate an IEC intervention anywhere on the African continent. It suggests that, in spite of a national policy of health care sector decentralization (Kyaddondo and Whyte, 2003), most of the significant interactions between MRC staff and Ugandan officialdom occurred not at the district level but at the national level. Admittedly, funds at the district level are limited (Kapiriri et al., 2003), so only limited changes to policy or practice could have taken place, but the principle still applies that with effectively no input into, or awareness of a study at the district level, no action is likely to be forthcoming as a result of its findings.

At the national and international levels, things were more complicated, with three main reasons explaining the study's lack of impact. These were: (i) the length of time it took to complete the work and then publish the study's findings, (ii) the complexity of the findings, and (iii) the fact that people tended to take the findings to support a position that they already held.

With respect to the first of these reasons, the MIT was conceived in 1992, but the results were not published until 2003. At the time of publication, therefore, the MIT had existed as an entity for literally half as long as the AIDS epidemic itself, and the cutting-edge-research questions about HIV prevention that initially inspired it had simply become outdated by the time the results emerged. This is not to suggest that the issue of how best to reduce new HIV infections was no longer relevant, but rather that by the early-mid 2000s, other issues—not least a rapidly growing interest in ART—had taken precedence in policy makers' minds.

Furthermore, Uganda in the early 1990s was in the throes of one of the world's most devastating AIDS epidemics, with an estimated 1.5 million Ugandans HIV-infected in 1990 and prevalence rates among pregnant women in some areas as high as 39 percent (ACP, 1991). Finding empirically grounded ways to reduce HIV incidence was clearly a priority at that stage. But by 2003, Uganda had become established as *the* African AIDS success story, with well-documented reductions in HIV prevalence across much of the country. No policy maker had any interest in threatening that hard-earned and lucrative position by suggesting that the IEC intervention approach adopted by the MIT—which, in tone if not in intensity, broadly reflected the approach taken by the country as a whole—had been misguided or ineffective. Thus they were very happy to extrapolate the MRC's interpretation of the findings to the national context—"don't change anything, because you're already doing the right things"—and to keep on with business as usual.

One of the main—if, perhaps, rather obvious—lessons to be learned from this is to ensure that intervention trials are conceived, conducted, and the results analyzed, published, and disseminated as fast as is practicable. A study that aims to follow up people for 4 years or so should ideally not take 11 years to complete; and if it does, it is not unreasonable if the results are not then taken very seriously by policy makers. The epidemiological and policy landscapes will inevitably have changed by the time the results are published, and they are therefore most unlikely even to enter the "policy primeval soup" (Kingdon, cited in Evans and Davies, 1999:379), let alone to have any substantive impact on the policy process.

A second issue that reduced the policy impact of the study findings was that, in the words of the WHO consultant referred to in the text, "the results were all over the place." The primary outcome measure—HIV incidence—naturally dominated discussion, and the fact that even the MRC's analysis team initially struggled to explain the lack of impact on this goes some way to explain in turn why so few people in the Ugandan Ministry of Health understood what had been found. These were difficult findings, in stark contrast to the easily grasped 42 percent reduction in HIV incidence found in the Mwanza trial, a finding that brought about a direct impact on a number of countries' clinic-based HIV prevention strategies (Philpott et al., 2002).

Among international-level AIDS epidemiologists, this very same complexity was seized upon as a golden opportunity to enhance their understanding of the dynamics of HIV transmission—even if the eventual outcome of their deliberations did not actually contribute to any sort of policy debate. As one of those quoted above explained, "this to me is like a real-life example of how incrementally you get a better and better sense of approaching reality, approaching what's true. I just think that the next trial or big bit of information clears the picture a bit." And indeed, the epidemiological picture that arose out of Masaka built directly on that which had emerged out of Mwanza and Rakai.

But this incremental growth in knowledge, and the insights it brought about, also highlight the fact that the response to Mwanza in 1995 was, in hindsight, far too optimistic and simplistic. When the Mwanza trial was published in the *Lancet*, the editorial title published alongside it ("STD control for HIV prevention—it works!") was "true," at least within the context of what was known then. But such a breathless title could never be written today, given what has been learned in the meantime. When the disappointing Rakai results were published four years later, the accompanying commentary piece took great pains to explain the importance of the maturity of an AIDS epidemic in relation to the likely effectiveness of an STD control strategy for HIV prevention: the younger an epidemic, the more effective STD control would be. Hence, in Rakai's relatively mature epidemic, the strategy had been ineffective (Hitchcock and Fransen, 1999). Then, after the Masaka trial results were published, the accompanying commentary took the argument back one step further still, pointing out that this had been the "right trial at the wrong time," and that "rigorous evaluation of promising interventions should be encouraged early on when HIV incidence is rising and high-risk groups are readily identifiable" (Stephenson and Cowan, 2003:633). In other words, the level of belief in what could be accomplished receded as the knowledge base grew. After Mwanza, the belief was that STD control "works!"; after Rakai, it was held to be effective only early on in an AIDS epidemic; and after Masaka, STD control and community-based IEC could only be *shown* to be effective early on in an AIDS epidemic. Since none of East, Central, or Southern Africa was still experiencing an immature AIDS epidemic by that stage, the Masaka results were therefore of pure academic interest and no more.

In sum, the impact of the Masaka results was reduced both by their inherent complexity, and also because, when placed into their historical and epidemiological context, they were rendered so watered-down and insubstantial as to be of no real use to policy makers. Thus, to counter the optimistic view of the epidemiologist quoted above—that more knowledge inexorably brings us closer to the "truth"—it could equally be argued that this very same move toward the truth works as a hindrance to action. An epidemiologist may see the additional complexity as an exciting challenge to untangle and, indeed, professional knowledge of the dynamics of HIV transmission may now be more complete than it was prior to Masaka. But most people, policy makers among them, are likely to see the complexity within that knowledge base as an impenetrable web; and the easiest thing to do then is to ignore it altogether.

The third major problem for the Masaka trial results relates to the second, and was summed up by one of the UNAIDS officials I interviewed: "Where you have an absence of a clear, single finding, people will go off and make selective use of data . . . everybody will walk away with what they want." None of what is presented above suggests that the MIT changed anybody's mind about anything. Rather, it was interpreted to support a wide variety of pre-existing opinions, hopes, or beliefs. At all three levels, the study and its results were seen in the context of how people already saw the world: the reaction of everyone who encountered it was defined by their own professional or personal context.

Taking the three levels in turn: after much deliberation, international-level AIDS epidemiologists achieved a consensus about the inherent value of STD control, using the Masaka trial as supporting evidence, irrespective of its impact on HIV incidence. STD control was something they already valued highly, and aspects of the Masaka trial results were used to support this position, with the inconvenient findings about genital herpes (which did not fit the argument) being quietly left out of the discussion.

People in the Ugandan Ministry of Health, who had no wish to challenge the country's broadly successful HIV prevention status quo, saw the study as largely irrelevant, although its results were reportedly used to provide a firmer rationale for the ongoing policy of STD control in the context of general reproductive health. There was an overall sense that the need for research in the area of HIV prevention was overstated by the donor community, and these national-level policy makers were satisfied to base their judgments regarding at least behavioral HIV prevention strategy on what they felt to be straightforward common sense.

At the local level in Masaka, there appeared to be a strong belief among many of the former volunteer field workers—as implementers of the IEC intervention—that their HIV prevention work had been useful and valuable. Their comments to me regarding the effectiveness of their work referred not to the post-trial feedback, presented by the MRC at village meetings, which could easily have been misunderstood to indicate that the intervention had been successful.[24] Rather they spoke of the value inherent in their approach to community education. "We went to the people direct," one said. "People are so much interested in those drama shows," said another. In other words, they believed that what they were doing was appropriate and correct, and they used this as evidence that it must have been effective. Thus they were satisfied about their positive contribution to the community.

This leads directly to my concluding point, a moment of self-reflection, since most of what I took away myself from the study was also based on my personal and professional position. My own frustration about the trial results had been based on the fact that so much work had gone into the project but there had been so little to show for it at the end. I therefore found myself looking for any crumb of evidence to convince myself that my own five-year investment in the venture had not been entirely in vain. Such a crumb emerged during further analysis of the trial dataset, which showed that as many as 88 percent of the men interviewed in the study communities said they had been to at least one of the IEC activities during the previous 12 months, with 80 percent of the women saying the same

(Quigley et al., 2004:2058). I felt very satisfied that so many people—these figures translated to over 50,000 people across Masaka—had directly encountered the work of the IEC section, and that at least they had learned something and perhaps thought about HIV prevention in relation to their own lives. I therefore took what I wanted from the study to suit my own position—to convince myself that in some respects all my work had not been for nothing—just as almost everyone else who had been touched by the trial took it one way or another to justify or support something that they already believed, or wanted to believe.

What Has Guided AIDS Control Policy in Uganda?

Introduction

The idea for this book arose in my mind out of two troubling and related issues. Nelson Mandela had spoken passionately at the Durban International AIDS Conference in 2000, about a set of HIV prevention strategies whose value and effectiveness he said could not be disputed. These were precisely the strategies we had evaluated within the Masaka Intervention Trial (MIT)—promoting a delay in sexual debut for young people, zero-grazing, condoms, and treating STDs. But we had found these strategies to have no effect on HIV incidence. My first concern, therefore, was that there was a strong and widespread belief that certain approaches to HIV prevention were "known" to be effective, but our findings suggested—at least within the context of Masaka in the mid-late 1990s—that these very approaches were actually *in*effective. My second worry was that these findings were not taken to heart by policy makers or HIV prevention practitioners either in Uganda or elsewhere in Africa. Nothing changed, and business continued as usual. This indicated to me that scientific findings that went counter to the status quo were simply ignored by a billion-dollar international AIDS juggernaut with too much momentum and perhaps too many vested interests to countenance a change in direction. Certainly there could be no admission that perhaps the standard HIV prevention package used throughout Africa was misguided. To paraphrase Nelson Mandela, it seemed to me that politics had taken primacy over science.

In fact, I was wrong. Chapter 6 has shown that there was no such grand conspiracy, and that our science had been set aside for rather more mundane reasons. The MIT did have all the right qualifications for influencing policy—in terms of methodological approach (notwithstanding the critiques of the randomized controlled trial, as given in Chapter 2);

the importance of the question being asked; and the combination of senior Ugandan and expatriate staff members, most of whom were known within the Ministry of Health. But its downfall was the complexity and, at first sight, the counterintuitive nature of some of the results, as well as the fact that over a decade had elapsed since the idea for the study had been conceived. What had been cutting-edge in the early 1990s simply no longer had the same resonance by the time the results came out 11 years later. Where the Mwanza STD trial results had been met with near-euphoria in 1995, and the Rakai STD study findings had brought about dismay in 1998, Masaka emerged onto this increasingly complex epidemiological field in 2003 as a damp squib.

Through understanding this, and through acknowledging the lessons it teaches for AIDS research in general, I have resolved in my mind the problem that initially set me on the path to write this book. In the process, I have also examined the wider relationship between evidence and Uganda's generally successful HIV control policies over the course of the AIDS epidemic. In this final chapter, I will therefore seek both to synthesize this material, and to identify the factors that have guided AIDS control policy in Uganda.

The Myth of Evidence-Based Policy Making

There has been ongoing official rhetoric on the role of evidence in AIDS policy making in Uganda for at least ten years now. This has corresponded with the simultaneous emergence in the global literature of the concept of evidence-based health policy making, which itself appeared a few years after evidence-based medicine became the dominant paradigm for clinical practice in the early 1990s. It would therefore be reasonable to expect evidence to have played an important role in defining AIDS control policy at least in recent years; and it would not be entirely unreasonable to expect that it may have played some role even before the term became formally adopted into policy parlance.

But one of the points that emerged during my investigations was the contradiction that exists between the public rhetoric of Ugandan health policy makers on this subject and what they say in private. Privately, several of my respondents in the Ministry of Health argued that the need for research has been somewhat overstated by the donor community, adding that many of the policies they have put forward have been based on common sense and on their knowledge of what has been practically and culturally feasible. More specifically, one of those who has been most publicly vocal about the evidence-based nature of policy making in Uganda conceded to me in his Ministry office that AIDS research and AIDS policy in the country are "not now linked as well as they should be. Most research in the past has been basic and has had little to do with policy." One reason for this is that most AIDS research in Uganda has historically been instigated, led, and funded by non-Ugandans. This means both that it has often focused on issues other than those deemed to be of critical national importance, and also that there has been very little national-level ownership of the results. From a linkages perspective—as discussed in Chapter 2—one could therefore argue that there has in fact been a *missing* link between research and policy.

This point could also be taken one step further. The material presented in this book shows that there has been an evidence void on critical aspects of AIDS control over the course of the entire epidemic. No conclusive, unambiguous body of evidence actually existed on most of the strategic issues relevant to AIDS control and, as such, a truly evidence-based policy process would therefore not have been possible, irrespective of policy makers' public statements. This has applied both to HIV prevention— since the evidence concerning appropriate and effective strategies is both limited and ambiguous—as well as to the scaling up of ART provision, for which there was only evidence from small-scale pilot studies to support the suggestion that national-level provision was feasible. If one takes the analogy of a bridge designed to link research and policy, one sees that it is not just the bridge that is missing. There is also hardly any substantive and relevant research for one end of any such bridge to reach out to, which leaves just an evidence-free policy, standing alone.

The phrase "substantive and relevant" is critical here. I am not arguing that no evidence has existed, or that evidence has played no role in identifying the need for changes in policy over the course of the Ugandan epidemic. It is clear, for example, that the initial epidemiological studies— which established that AIDS was present in Uganda, and which also identified high-risk groups—proved invaluable in establishing the need for AIDS control in the first place. Even so, connecting the evidence with the policy makers did not happen automatically. David Serwadda, first author of the breakthrough 1985 *Lancet* paper about AIDS in Masaka, complained to me that there was initially a distinct lack of interest within the Ministry of Health about the findings, and that he had to be "proactive" in bringing them to people's attention. The difficult link between evidence and policy makers was also bridged by the surveillance data that showed ever-increasing HIV prevalence rates in the late 1980s. This was used to convince President Museveni in 1991 of the urgent need to enhance HIV prevention activities.

But while the studies clearly showed the need for action, their very nature—descriptive, cross-sectional sero-surveys—meant that they could not identify exactly what sort of action should be taken. As sociologist

Maxine Ankrah pointed out early in the epidemic, there has been "too much epidemiology, too little social science" (Ankrah, 1989:267) in the study of AIDS in Uganda, as well as more widely in Africa. The relative proportions of epidemiology and social scientific work may since have shifted slightly in favor of social science but a body of evidence has nonetheless been produced, which is weighted inappropriately toward those areas that can be measured, leaving aside those that by their very nature cannot. Such a "restrictive" (Nutbeam, 1999:100) and "reductionist" (Bonell, 2002:386) epidemiological evidence base is unable to capture the complexity inherent in the essential social determinants of, for example, HIV prevention or adherence to ART. Its potential for defining policies is therefore inevitably limited. To quote Albert Einstein again: "Not everything that can be counted counts, and not everything that counts can be counted."

In the context of the evolving HIV prevention policy of the 1980s and 1990s, this meant that there was no empirical basis for arguing that any new policy should promote abstinence, faithfulness, or condom use, or a combination thereof. In other words, while recognition of the need for an HIV prevention policy may have been evidence-based, the exact form of the policy that emerged was not. Thus there are different layers regarding which aspect of a policy may be evidence-based and which may not be. And, as has been shown throughout the book, in the absence of relevant, unambiguous evidence, it is all too easy to make either selective use or a creative interpretation of what there is in support of pre-existing or ideological policy positions.

It is important to note that actors at both the international and national levels have been prone to doing this. There are several such examples, including the use of the pepper evidence by the Catholic authorities to "prove" that condoms were not effective against HIV, and therefore that they should not be promoted; the evidence used by former U.S. Secretary of State Colin Powell to argue for an "empirically-based" ABC strategy that had no condom component; the evidence used by Janet Museveni and the U.S. evangelical Christians during the PEPFAR Congressional debates suggesting that abstinence had led to the fall in HIV prevalence in Uganda; and the evidence of individuals in Africa who showed very high levels of adherence to ARVs in pilot programs, thereby seeking to demonstrate to the doubters that adherence in Africa would not be a problem.

The policies that followed from each of these assertions may therefore have been evidence-based, in the sense that their proponents had used evidence to support them; and some of these individuals may have sincerely believed that the evidence they were using was watertight and definitive. However, the evidence used in each of these cases could in fact be interpreted in different ways according to the ideology of the person interpreting it. Collectively, therefore, these examples show the importance of always being wary of "agendas that go beyond AIDS"—as Harvard University's Ted Green has phrased it—whenever evidence in support of a given position is being presented. Returning to the bridge analogy, we now see that our "evidence-free" policy is not actually standing alone. Rather, it is linked by a bridge in another direction altogether, to ideology. The relationship between ideology and policy will be discussed further below.

Related to this are the changing ways in which a given piece of evidence can be used. Evidence can be produced, for example, with an explicitly political agenda, such as the ART pilot studies that were conducted in order to demonstrate that ART provision in developing countries was feasible. This evidence was then used with great success as an advocacy tool in support of global ART scale-up. But evidence can also be produced for ostensibly more neutral purposes—such as the national Demographic and Health Surveys of 1989 and 1995—and then it can be turned for political purposes at a later date. Individually, these cross-sectional DHS surveys sought to provide a snapshot of demographic and health-related issues in Uganda; and together, they were able to identify trends in, among many other things, sexual behavior. At the time of publication, they were considered to be interesting, if not of global concern. But increasing international awareness in the early 2000s of Uganda's success in reducing HIV prevalence and incidence subsequently reawakened interest in these datasets—there was virtually no other comparable evidence available from the period—and they became the core evidence around which the highly political ABC debate then revolved. Such unexpected linkages across time demonstrate how evidence can be produced for one purpose, and yet it can subsequently be used for something quite different.

Aside from such cases of what could be described as the opportunistic interpretation and use of evidence, it is clear, therefore, that strategic AIDS control policies in Uganda—those concerned with the broad approaches to reducing HIV incidence and those focused on how best or indeed whether to scale up provision of ART—have not been evidence-based. As of 2005, even the methodological approach standing at the summit of the evidence hierarchy—the mighty Randomized Controlled Trial—had played hardly any role in formulating policy for one of Africa's most innovative and effective national AIDS control efforts.[1] But official rhetoric notwithstanding, this is not an entirely unexpected conclusion. The literature review in Chapter 2 described a generic theory of policy development that suggested that there are a number of factors that may play a role during each phase of the policy process. Evidence is only one of these, and indeed some authors have gone so far as to argue that "[evidence derived from] research has, in fact, little impact on policy making" (Poulos and Zwi, 2005:429). This book has therefore confirmed that what is to be found elsewhere in the general process of policy development also applies specifically to AIDS control policy in Uganda. But an additional point has emerged here, in the form of the divergence between the rhetoric and the reality. Official rhetoric maintains that AIDS policy formulation in the country is evidence-based. However, not only is this overstating the case, but such rhetoric is rarely, if ever, challenged, thus allowing the perpetuation of a myth.

Why is this so? Tilley and Laycock (2000:213) argue that "rooting policy in evidence has all the appeal of motherhood and apple pie—the rhetoric is cheap and easy." Such "cheap and easy" rhetoric can have great benefits. Uganda has used the deepening and largely donor-inspired interest in the concept of evidence-based policy making adeptly to its own advantage. As shown in the previous chapters, the country has attained a great deal of legitimacy in the eyes of the international community through its success in tackling AIDS—and the country's adoption into its public lexicon of the principle of evidence-based policy making has only strengthened that legitimacy. The reasons for the public rhetoric are therefore clear.

As for why the rhetoric remains unchallenged, one could argue that policy makers have effectively painted themselves into a corner with their ongoing claims of evidence-based AIDS control policies. With their credibility at stake, they are unlikely now to admit publicly that, at least with respect to the strategic policies for AIDS control, and at least up until 2005, this was not the case. Likewise, since funders of scientific work usually include a section in their grant proposal forms asking how the evidence produced will have practical or policy implications, researchers are also unlikely to concede that their work rarely does so. With both groups having such a clear interest in maintaining the myth of evidence-based policy making, any such challenge is unlikely to come from the inside. Furthermore, even if the literature suggests that the link is tenuous at best in policy settings throughout the world, and therefore that this is by no means a purely Ugandan phenomenon, there may be a natural reluctance to attract the sort of opprobrium that Justin Parkhurst received in 2002 when he offered his critique of the epidemiological evidence that had shaped Uganda's reputation as an AIDS success story (Parkhurst, 2002).

While recognizing this possible hazard, I would argue nonetheless for a downgrading of the term "evidence-based policy making" for AIDS control in Uganda. The combined wisdom of two of my respondents provides the starting point for an alternative way of thinking about this issue. The political science lecturer at Makerere University explained that "policy is ultimately driven by values, and values are not shaped by research. Policies are value-based, not evidence-based." Meanwhile the top-level UNAIDS official in Geneva asserted that "I'm a believer in evidence-informed policy, not in evidence-based policy." Both these comments recognize that political and other factors—including individual histories, experiences, beliefs, prejudices, competencies, and skills, as well as communication with colleagues and other informal linkages (see, for example, Bowen and Zwi, 2005)—play a central role in the policy process. They also avoid giving a misleading rhetorical primacy to evidence.

We are still left, however, with a situation in which a large amount of AIDS research is conducted in Uganda, quantities of evidence are produced and published, but then the policy process, the nature of the evidence, or a combination of the two results in no real changes in policy or practice. This inevitably begs the question: What is the point of doing such work in the first place? Not only is AIDS research expensive—and, for many study participants, positively intrusive—but in the words of a speaker during a debate at a conference that I attended in 2003, if our work is not practically relevant to some aspect of AIDS control, are we not "just playing fun mind games"? With over 40 million people currently HIV-infected worldwide— of whom around 1 million live in Uganda alone—this is a distasteful and disturbing image, one truly evocative of fiddling while Rome burns.

I do not want to strike a nihilist note here, and I am not suggesting at all that AIDS research can serve no purpose. Research does have a role to play, but the problems must first be recognized if they are to be addressed, and researchers themselves need to acknowledge that many of the potential solutions lie in their court.

For example, it is essential that they focus, through a multidisciplinary approach, more on the issues that are likely to be directly useful to policy makers, as well as on those that are relevant at the local level, where any services coming out of the research would eventually be based. The fact that so much of the AIDS research conducted in Uganda has had such limited significance, either for policy or for practice, points to wasted opportunities and wasted resources.

Researchers also have a responsibility to inform policy makers about the issues that they may not know that they need to know about. While they may feel that the importance of research has been overstated, several Ugandan Ministerial officials were nonetheless concerned by their lack of knowledge about AIDS research in the country, both in terms of aware- ness about ongoing studies as well as in terms of having access to the findings. Just because evidence is low on the list of influences to which policy makers are subjected does not mean that research findings do not interest them.

In addition, much could be gained by researchers reflecting more on policy-making theory, since it appears that they often have a somewhat simplistic, linear view of the process. As discussed in Chapter 2, Walt et al.

(2003:12) describe the global policy adoption of syndromic STD management as "diffuse, iterative and looped"; and while this portrayal was applied to just one particular policy, parallels can surely also be drawn in relation to the development of many others. Recognition of the inherent complexity of health policy making should, ideally, stimulate researchers to look out more actively for possible entry points into the process, through which they may then contribute, either nationally or internationally. Kingdon's (1984) three-stream model—including the problem stream, the policy stream, and the politics stream—could be a useful conceptual tool here. He argues that issues join the policy primeval soup to compete with other issues for attention and funding only when there is a confluence of the three streams. But in a world of (theoretically) evidence-based policy making, a fourth stream could also be added—the evidence stream—through which researchers could aim at actively creating windows of opportunity for influencing the process.

As Anna Donald argues through a powerful analogy, it is essential to keep striving toward the goal of producing more fully evidence-informed policies, regardless of the difficulties: "As a form of governance, democracy is also difficult and imperfect, and terrible things happen that shouldn't— corruption, war, poverty, and crime. Yet that does not mean that we yearn to return to less questioning and more precarious forms of governance such as oligarchies and dictatorships, however benign" (Donald, 2001:279). Similarly, evidence-based policies are an ideal that may never be fully achieved, but which are worth continually working toward nonetheless. One condition for achieving this goal is to identify the missing links that exist—between individual actors and between the two professions of research and policy making—and then seek to build bridges to link them. Unless and until these links are made, other, more ideologically driven influences will inevitably continue to take precedence.

Ideological Context and Pragmatic Choices

If AIDS research has not played an important role in defining either policy or practice for AIDS control in Uganda, how, then, has the process actually worked? Ideological influences have clearly been a significant driving force, but it is self-evident that before any decision—ideological or otherwise—regarding the direction of AIDS control activities can even be contemplated, the stage must first be set by an essential prerequisite: recognition of the need to act.

This recognition took place at the national level in 1986, in the mind of President Museveni. Museveni had seen the catastrophe of AIDS at first hand as he fought through Rakai and Masaka, and he had also learned from

Fidel Castro that his own army—which he relied on to keep him in power in a highly volatile situation—was heavily affected. In this, he was unique among his East African presidential peers, none of whom had recently fought their way to power, and none of whom had personally witnessed the decimation of entire villages by AIDS. But Museveni also had the very pragmatic insight that there was more to gain by action than there was to lose. Indeed, there was nothing to lose. Uganda's economy in 1986 could surely sink no lower, and there were no tourists or investors to scare away by admitting to a serious AIDS epidemic. Consequently, the decision to act was made, and his government adopted an open AIDS policy that year, both to attract international technical and financial assistance, and also to encourage a robust and innovative national and local-level response.

Through grasping the reality of the country's ongoing, chronic emergency, and the consequent imperative to act, this open policy has implicitly facilitated every decision on AIDS control since then. It has also stimulated an extremely dynamic national response over the years by actively welcoming foreign intervention, and has thereby established itself within what could be described as a path-dependent process. This can be seen as a series of "self-reinforcing sequences characterized by the formation and long-term reproduction of a given institutional pattern" (Mahoney, 2000:508). Uganda was already being internationally lauded for its openness about AIDS in the late 1980s, which served to attract ever more foreign agencies and financing into the country over the 1990s and 2000s. By thus continually reinforcing this particular institutional pattern, success has fed success, and President Museveni's early pragmatic recognition of the need to act against AIDS has paid off handsomely.

With the ongoing need to act established, ideology has provided the broad context in which all subsequent decisions have been made, and has thereby played a crucial role in determining the nature of those decisions. Ideology is an elusive concept,[2] and in order to embrace the political, cultural, and moral concerns that have featured extensively throughout the course of the Ugandan AIDS epidemic, I have taken the following definition here: "The promotion and legitimation of the interests of [a] social group in the face of opposing interests" (Eagleton, 2007:29). The word "opposing" is central to the discussion, since opposition from some quarters both to change and to the status quo has characterized most of the events portrayed in this book. And with this constant opposition of views, there have also been regular shifts in the dominant ideology of the day, as one social group dominates the scene for a period, before eventually being pushed aside by another. Thus the nature of the decisions has also changed.

Discussions over strategies for HIV prevention have always had a strong ideological streak, since the topic intrinsically concerns how, the extent to which, and with whom people have sex. These are issues about which politicians, religious leaders, and international donors have expressed clear and often uncompromising views over the course of the epidemic. But there has been an ideological ebb and flow in the international-level debates, and this has brought about shifts and even reversals in the ideological context on which the national-level decisions regarding HIV prevention have then been made. This is not at all to suggest that international agendas have had hegemony over Ugandan policies, but they have undoubtedly exerted a strong influence.

For example, in the early days of the Ugandan epidemic, a strong and pervasive Catholic influence combined with a morally conservative population to provide the dominant ideology. Over the 1990s, a foreign ideology—intent on the promotion of condoms—increasingly dominated the scene in Uganda, though not without considerable resistance. And as PEPFAR appeared in 2003, with its promise of tens of millions of strings-attached dollars, there was a return to a more conservative moral ideology for HIV prevention. This shifting in the leading ideological position of the day stimulated a series of political decisions in Kampala that continually amended and updated the national HIV prevention strategy.

The global move toward scale-up of ART provision was also fraught with ideological conflict. The main protagonists on one side of the divide were an alliance of activists, advocate-scientists, and the Big Men of finance and politics. They were appalled by the inequities brought about by these very expensive, life-saving drugs that were accessible to AIDS patients in wealthy countries, but—throughout the 1990s and very early 2000s—which were almost totally absent in Africa. This was morally unacceptable, they felt, and it simply had to be challenged. The powerhouse on the other side of the ideological divide was comprised of the pharmaceutical companies that made the drugs. They saw things primarily from a business perspective, and were very reluctant to reduce the price of their products, arguing both that their shareholders would not accept it, and also that reducing prices would decrease profits, which in turn would undermine future possibilities for pharmaceutical research and development.

This bitter ideological battle was effectively won by the principle of equity. The Big Men and their activist supporters celebrated as the drug prices came down, and huge quantities of donor money emerged in order to buy them for distribution to African patients. Consequently, by 2003 or shortly thereafter, ART was irreversibly on the national policy agendas of Uganda and every other heavily affected country in the world.

It has therefore been within particular ideological contexts that decisions have been made about the course of action for AIDS control policies and practices, and the decisions have generally been made on a pragmatic basis. I am not using the term "pragmatic" here in its philosophical sense.[3] Rather I am taking it as defined through its standard, everyday usage: "a practical and realistic way of dealing with things" (OED, 2005:798). My argument here is that within the ideological context of the day, decisions have tended to be made practically and realistically. They have been based either on what is seen to be feasible and likely to work—lack of evidence notwithstanding—or on what will attract money or political capital, or both.

I also argue that the evolving, pragmatic strategic course for HIV prevention and the scale-up of ART provision has invariably been set by the primary individual actor, President Museveni himself. He has had unparalleled access to the key players at both the national and international levels, and this has given him a unique authority to decide which approach for a given problem appeared to be most advantageous—both for him and for Uganda. He has not always moved as his personal ideological convictions would have preferred, choosing instead directions that appeared likely to bring other practical and political benefits.

For example, in the early epidemic, it would not have been pragmatic—that is, neither practical nor realistic—to promote condoms as a means of preventing HIV. This particular approach would have been perceived as unacceptably licentious by many Ugandans, and would have served only to alienate them, thereby undermining the rest of the national HIV prevention program. At that stage and within this ideological context, therefore, promoting only zero-grazing and abstinence, as sanctioned by President Museveni, was an eminently pragmatic approach. But with the international prevailing wind starting to blow firmly in a pro-condom direction during the 1990s, Museveni saw that there was more to gain than to lose—again, both for him and for Uganda—by accepting this evolving status quo. For entirely pragmatic reasons, and even though it went against his own ideological preference, the condom policy was therefore gradually liberalized. Through this, Museveni maintained his status as an African AIDS leader in the eyes of the international community, and he also ensured the continued flow of much-needed financing into the country.

Things are not so clear-cut after 2003, when the moral and political battle over how to spend the $3 billion allocated by PEPFAR for HIV prevention ended with a return to the ideological ground on which Museveni felt much more comfortable. Condoms had been forced off center stage by the world's most powerful international donor, which required aspiring recipient nations such as Uganda to target condom promotion only for high-risk groups, not for the general population, and certainly not for young people. But the response in Uganda was confused, with the Ministry of Health finally publishing its pro-condom policy, Museveni publicly denouncing condoms at the 2004 International AIDS Conference in Bangkok, and condoms being withdrawn from shelves across the country. Some people claimed the withdrawal was for technical reasons, while others said it was because of American ideological pressure. But whatever the reason, an acute nationwide shortage of condoms was the result, and Museveni had—very pragmatically—further endeared himself to a U.S. administration that had recently provided Uganda with her first tranche of PEPFAR funding, to the tune of $91 million.

With regard to the scale-up or ART provision, once the ideological battle had been won by the Big Men and their activist allies, the issues requiring attention were no longer ideological, but were instead entirely pragmatic. The work of Peter Mugyenyi at the Joint Clinical Research Centre, as well as the facilities that had been engaged in the Drug Access Initiative, had shown that if large-scale, equitable ART provision were to be feasible, it would have to be free for patients. This meant that donors would have to cover the costs of every patient taken on, in perpetuity. What, therefore, was the most "practical and realistic" way to ensure this for a putative national ART program?

The unrequested arrival into Uganda of the U.S.-based AIDS Healthcare Foundation in late 2001 brought matters to a head. AHF's ambitious plan for Uganda was to set up a system with a guarantee to provide free treatment for life for every patient they took on. Through this, the problem of sustainability would be resolved, at least in their Uganda Cares clinics. But many of President Museveni's advisors felt that the proposal could turn out to be the thin end of an unsustainable wedge, by stimulating a demand for free ART throughout the country that could overwhelm an already struggling health service. This, they argued, was not pragmatic—it was neither practical nor realistic, and could not feasibly be realized—and they therefore strongly opposed it.

Museveni himself, however, had a different vision of pragmatism. He saw the many benefits that would accrue if Uganda Cares were to succeed: benefits to the care and conditions of Ugandans living with AIDS, to Uganda's reputation, and, by proxy, to himself. He doubtless also anticipated the way that Uganda Cares would act as a catalyst for larger-scale free ART provision in the country. But rather than seeing this as the thin end of an unsustainable wedge, he saw that the pragmatic option was instead to go with the global wind that was just then changing in the direction of free ART provision. Therefore, he threw his full support behind Uganda Cares, going so far as personally to facilitate the accreditation of their first clinic, in Masaka. Where the pragmatism of Museveni's advisors led them to conclude that "this cannot work," the pragmatism of Museveni himself could be characterized as a determination to "make this work, and make this work for us."

I have argued here that three factors at the international and national levels have been primarily responsible for shaping Uganda's historically successful strategy for AIDS control. The first of these—a prerequisite for the others—has been *recognition of the need to act*. Decisions on the course of action to be taken have then been heavily influenced by the dominant international or national *ideological context* of the day, with *pragmatism* within that ideological context ultimately defining the eventual policy decision. Furthermore, evidence has, in many cases, been interpreted explicitly to support these decisions.

A final note is also due here regarding the local level, which has been conspicuously absent from this multilevel discussion. The objective of AIDS control efforts is, obviously, to provide local communities with effective prevention and treatment services. Everything described in this book has had this as its ultimate stated aim, even if the field of play may be littered with an array of other, unrelated agendas. It is ironic, therefore, that the people with the most to gain and the most to lose—those living at the local level—have essentially no voice in deciding which sort of services they will receive. Decisions are made on their behalf in Kampala and further afield, and they become the silent recipients of whatever it is decided should come their way. From a multilevel perspective, all the arrows from the national and international levels point toward them, and they have little or no opportunity to provide input into any of the decisions. In this sense, ordinary people at the local level represent a *non*-influence, a dead end in the process.

The words of one of my respondents in rural Masaka provide food for thought in this regard. "The common man," he told me, "feels that he is the project of the higher people. The common man here *feeds* the higher people." Within the framework outlined above, those of us who earn our living studying, making policy, or designing AIDS control services for people at the local level must continually ask ourselves what more we can do to ensure that their needs and interests are taken into account. The "common man" should not merely be "the project of the higher people." He and his family should be active participants in the process, and their voices must be heard.

Appendix: Multilevel Timeline of Key Events

	International	National (Uganda)	Local (Masaka-Rakai area)
1978	• Alma Ata Declaration: "Health for all by the year 2000."	• Idi Amin invades Kagera Salient, Tanzania, and provokes war.	
1979		• Idi Amin ousted.	• Tanzanian troops respond to invasion, crossing into Uganda from Kagera. • Masaka town razed by Tanzanian troops—chaos, looting, and rape.
1980			
1981	• World's first published report of AIDS, in United States.	• Civil War ongoing.	
1982		• Civil War ongoing.	• Eighty-four cases of Slim registered in Masaka's Kitovu Hospital.
1983	• Virus that causes AIDS discovered by Luc Montagnier—named LAV. • Recognition of AIDS in Zaire.	• Civil War ongoing. • Anne Bailey speaks in Kampala of an increase in Atypical Kaposi's sarcoma in Zambia.	
1984	• "Another" AIDS virus discovered by Robert Gallo—named HTLV-III.	• Civil War ongoing. • Wilson Carswell establishes that HTLV-III exists in Uganda.	• November: first official report of Slim in Rakai sent to Kampala, no action taken. • December: article about Slim in Rakai appears in the *Star* newspaper.

(Continued)

	International	*National (Uganda)*	*Local (Masaka-Rakai area)*
1985		• Civil War ongoing. • Slim the most common cause of death at Mulago national referral hospital in Kampala. • Ten percent of pregnant women attending Mulago HTLV-III-positive.	• February: investigative team from Ministry of Health concludes that Slim is typhoid. • October: seminal article published in the *Lancet* detailing Slim in Masaka. Slim and AIDS said to be different entities.
1986	• Consensus attained that LAV and HTLV-III are the same virus—renamed HIV.	• January: Yoweri Museveni takes power. • June: blood screening begins in Nsambya Hospital, Kampala. • October: national Committee for the Prevention and Control of AIDS established (precursor to AIDS Control Programme). Concept of zero-grazing introduced.	
1987	• Peter Piot argues for education as the "main thrust" for AIDS control worldwide. • AZT approved by the U.S. Food and Drug Administration for use against HIV.	• Donors' conference held, $7.4 million pledged.	• Kitovu Hospital starts screening blood for HIV.
1988		• AIDS awareness pamphlets, badges, and stickers being distributed; condoms not promoted. • Twenty-five percent of pregnant women attending Mulago hospital HIV-positive.	

(Continued)

International	National (Uganda)	Local (Masaka-Rakai area)
	• Headquarters established in Entebbe for UK-funded Medical Research Programme (MRC) on AIDS, and U.S.-funded Rakai Project. • The AIDS Support Organisation (TASO) founded in Kampala.	
1989 • Uganda already internationally recognized for its open AIDS policy. • International AIDS Conference in Montreal: recognition that most AIDS social and epidemiological research in Africa is descriptive, with insufficient attention to the evaluation of interventions.	• Ugandan singer Philly Lutaaya publicly declares his HIV-positive status. • National-level recognition that knowledge of AIDS does not always lead to behavior change. • National Catholic authorities confirm that condom use is "unacceptable." • Nationwide Demographic and Health Survey conducted.	• MRC established in rural Masaka—HIV prevalence estimated at 8 percent. • TASO opens its second office, in Masaka hospital.
1990 • International AIDS Conference in San Francisco: too much research in Africa is urban and convenience-based, ignoring heavily affected rural areas.	• Thirty-nine percent of pregnant women attending Mulago HIV-positive; 1.5 million Ugandans estimated to be infected with HIV.	• HIV prevalence rates in Rakai shown to vary from 12 percent in rural villages to 35 percent in main road trading centers.
1991 • Museveni speaks of "apocalypse" at International AIDS Conference in Florence. • Trial begins in Mwanza, Tanzania, to investigate effect of syndromic STD management on HIV incidence.	• Museveni agrees to permit "quiet" condom promotion. • Protector condoms make their Ugandan debut, with a modest, low-key advertising campaign. • USAID grants $12 million for HIV prevention.	

(Continued)

	International	*National (Uganda)*	*Local (Masaka-Rakai area)*
		• First Antiretroviral drugs (ARVs) provided at Joint Clinical Research Centre (JCRC) in Kampala. • Forty-four percent of STD patients attending Mulago hospital are HIV-positive.	
1992	• International NGOs release a Statement of Belief, affirming their *belief* in the value and effectiveness of behavior change for reducing new HIV infections. • WHO study suggests that 95 percent of 559 research projects identified in sub-Saharan Africa were "of no immediate relevance to the local populations."	• Uganda AIDS Commission (UAC) established. • HIV prevalence rates continue to rise at surveillance sites throughout the country. Rates in provincial antenatal surveillance sites range from 7 percent in the east to 30 percent in the southwest.	• Idea for Masaka Intervention Trial (MIT) conceived, to investigate the effect on HIV incidence of (i) a behavioral intervention and (ii) syndromic STD management. • Masaka reporting more clinical cases of AIDS than any district outside Kampala.
1993	• World Bank's World Development Report focuses on role of health in economic development.	• $73 million World Bank-funded six-year STI Project starts. • UAC: "a virtual explosion of [AIDS research] activity" has taken place, but it is uncoordinated.	• Ninety percent of patients on Kitovu Hospital medical wards suffering from AIDS-related conditions. • MIT study design finalized.
1994		• AIDS Control Programme (ACP) says there is a "noticeable decline in the rate of increase" in HIV prevalence in most of the country's sentinel surveillance sites.	• MRC study in preparation for MIT finds misconceptions about, and opposition to condoms. • Rakai project STD mass treatment study starts.

(Continued)

	International	National (Uganda)	Local (Masaka-Rakai area)
1995	• Mwanza STD trial results published: syndromic STD management found to reduce HIV incidence by 42 percent.	• UAC: "there are no articulated national policies on AIDS control." • First public suggestion of an overall decline in nationwide HIV prevalence. • Thirty-six percent of STD patients attending Mulago hospital are HIV-positive (down from 44 percent in 1991). • Nationwide Demographic and Health Survey conducted. • Median age for first sex found to be 16.3 among females and 17.3 among males.	• MIT surveys and interventions start in earnest.
1996	• Development of triple combination ARV therapy, or Highly Active Antiretroviral Therapy (HAART), for treating AIDS.	• Life Guard condoms appear on the market: eight U.S. cents buy three condoms. • JCRC treating 1,000 patients with Antiretroviral therapy (ART); patients on HAART pay $1,000 per month. • HIV prevalence rates at antenatal surveillance sites throughout the country now range from 2 percent to 15 percent.	
1997	• WHO Director General Hiroshi Nakajima warns that the new ARV regimens could draw policy makers' attention away from HIV prevention.	• Ugandan MP: "[A] comprehensive set of national [AIDS] policies is yet to be generated." • "Quiet" condom promotion scrapped; open promotion now permitted.	

(Continued)

	International	National (Uganda)	Local (Masaka-Rakai area)
		• Twelve hundred registered agencies implementing AIDS-related activities in Uganda. • Uganda joins the Drug Access Initiative (DAI) to increase access to ARVs.	
1998	• UNAIDS proclaims "Prevention works."	• Study finds national AIDS expenditure between 1989 and 1998 to be $180 million (= $1.80 per adult per year), of which 70 percent is covered by donors.	
1999		• Controversial Life Guard condom advertisement appears, depicting fun and sexy lifestyle. • Monthly cost of triple therapy has fallen to $500. • ACP estimates that 838,000 Ugandans have died from AIDS since the epidemic began.	• Rakai STD mass treatment study results published: no impact of intervention found.
2000	• Clinton administration describes AIDS as a threat to U.S. national security and to global stability. • International AIDS Conference in Durban: Mandela urges drastic action to fight AIDS.	• Median age for first sex found to have risen since 1995: now 16.6 among females and 18.5 among males. • HIV prevalence rates at antenatal surveillance sites throughout the country continue to fall. Now range from 1 percent to 12 percent.	• The number of condoms sold through MIT in the past four years is 1.5 million. • First indication of falling HIV incidence in any part of Africa found in MRC's Kyamulibwa general population cohort.

(Continued)

	International	*National (Uganda)*	*Local (Masaka-Rakai area)*
2001	• UN Special Session on HIV/AIDS (UNGASS) held. • In developing countries, 240,000 people receiving ART. • Cipla decides to produce generic ARVs, cutting the cost of triple therapy to $30 a month. • MSF starts pilot ART project in Khayelitsha, Cape Town.	• DAI transformed into a wider Accelerated Access Initiative. • Peter Mugyenyi illegally imports cheap generic ARVs and forces the government to permit importation of the drugs. • AHF holds conference on HIV care and support in Entebbe. Promises to open Uganda Cares ART clinic in Masaka. • Established national-level actors skeptical about Uganda Cares' chances of success.	• Masaka district chairman Vincent Ssempijja meets Michael Weinstein, President of the U.S.-based AIDS Healthcare Foundation (AHF).
2002	• Global Fund to Fight AIDS, Tuberculosis and Malaria founded. • Justin Parkhurst challenges the Uganda AIDS "success story." • Colin Powell advocates for a condom-free approach to HIV prevention. • International AIDS Conference in Barcelona: WHO Director General Gro Harlem Brundtland announces plans for massive global scale-up of ARV provision.	• The term "ABC" first used as a description of Uganda's approach to HIV prevention. • Drug resistance noted in 65 percent of patients from DAI. • Results-dissemination workshop held in Kampala for MRC's MIT: no impact from interventions found, policy makers advised to continue business as usual.	• Uganda Cares clinic opened in Masaka by First Lady Janet Museveni—promises free provision of ART and related services. Many people skeptical.

(Continued)

	International	National (Uganda)	Local (Masaka-Rakai area)
2003	• The U.S. President's Emergency Plan for AIDS Relief (PEPFAR) founded. Janet Museveni and U.S. Christian groups lobby for abstinence-only HIV prevention programs. • WHO launches '3 by 5'.	• Uganda receives $36 million from Global Fund for ARVs; announces its '3 by 5' target of 60,000 people to be on ART by end 2005. • National ART policy published. • Minister of Health Mike Mukula calls Uganda Cares a "proven initiative."	• After 12 months' work, Uganda Cares has established its operating procedures. One hundred patients are on its books, and the decision is made to scale up. • MRC's MIT study results published: no impact from interventions found.
2004	• International scientific consensus that the fall in HIV prevalence in Uganda was primarily due to a reduction in sexual partners. • International AIDS Conference in Bangkok: Museveni ambivalent about condoms. • Concerns felt in WHO headquarters about feasibility of '3 by 5.' • WHO recognizes Uganda Cares as best practice for ART provision.	• National Condom Policy and Strategy published: condoms to be "widely and openly promoted." • Uganda receives $91 million of PEPFAR money. • Value of condoms downplayed by State Minister for Information. • Ministry of Health withdraws tens of millions of condoms.	• Uganda Cares providing free ART to 802 patients—continues to expand.
2005	• The number of people receiving ART in developing countries is 1.3 million: '3 by 5' target missed by 1.7 million, but momentum growing nonetheless.	• Uganda exceeds '3 by 5' ART target: 67,000 people receiving treatment.	• Rakai study suggests primary cause of falling HIV prevalence was high mortality rather than falling HIV incidence.

Abbreviations: ACP, AIDS Control Programme; AHF, AIDS Healthcare Foundation; ART, Antiretroviral therapy; ARV, Antiretroviral drug; DAI, Drug Access Initiative; HAART, Highly Active Antiretroviral Therapy; JCRC, Joint Clinical Research Centre; MIT, Masaka Intervention Trial; MRC, Medical Research Council; PEPFAR, The U.S. President's Emergency Plan for AIDS Relief; TASO, The AIDS Support Organisation; UAC, Uganda AIDS Commission.

Some events took place across the boundaries of one level, but they are categorized into just one level here for the sake of clarity.

Notes

Chapter 1

1. HIV incidence refers to *new* cases of infection, and is usually presented as the percentage of the uninfected population that is infected in a given year. HIV prevalence, by contrast, represents the proportion of the whole population that is infected at any given time, and which therefore includes people who were infected some time ago. Although HIV incidence is technically much harder to measure than HIV prevalence—hence the long lapse in Uganda between demonstrating falls in prevalence and demonstrating falls in incidence—it is the key indicator for determining current trends in infection rates.

2. The study evaluated two HIV prevention interventions: (i) behavioral change, through what is known as Information, Education, and Communication (IEC), and (ii) the treatment of sexually transmitted diseases.

3. I use the term "AIDS control" to include both the prevention of HIV infection and the treatment of people who have AIDS. I finished my main fieldwork session in late 2004, but have followed up certain issues during a number of subsequent working visits to Uganda.

4. A classical example of presentism is given by Fischer (1970), who writes about the so-called Whig history. He describes how certain eighteenth- and nineteenth-century British historians wrote history in a way that used the past to validate their own political beliefs. This interpretation was presentist in the sense that it did not depict the past in what could be described as neutral historical context, but instead events were viewed through the lens of contemporary Whig (or, as the party evolved, Liberal) beliefs.

5. An emic perspective describes behaviors and understandings in terms meaningful (consciously or unconsciously) to the actor. By contrast, an etic account is a description of behavior in terms meaningful to the observer.

6. The former Masaka district has, over the years, been subdivided into these three districts, so they can be seen collectively as the greater Masaka region. This covers an area of 9,400 square kilometers, and had a population of slightly over 1.4 million people in 2002. Over 80 percent of these people live in rural areas (Uganda Bureau of Statistics, 2002a).

Chapter 2

1. Much qualitative social science draws from the idea that phenomena should be studied in their own context, and that macrolevel processes and structures are mediated through local-level actors. In this sense these studies implicitly adopt a multilevel perspective. The discussion here, however, focuses on those studies that have explicitly taken this approach, methodologically and/or analytically.

2. Critical medical anthropology was born out of a wish to politicize medical anthropology, and it took a clearly defined left-wing position.

3. Sixty-two out of 80 top officials appointed to the Ugandan Ministry of Health during a restructuring exercise in 1997/1998 were physicians (Jeppsson et al., 2005:315).

4. Epidemiology is defined as "the study of the distribution and determinants of disease frequency" (Hennekens and Buring, 1987:3).

5. Randomization is intended to eliminate the chance of bias in one or other of the groups and also to distribute demographic, behavioral, and/or clinical characteristics of study participants as evenly as possible between study groups so as to permit comparability (Hennekens and Buring, 1987:188).

6. Inductive inference works in the reverse direction: observations are made, on the basis of which a plausible hypothesis can then be developed in order to explain what has been seen.

7. The RCT did not constitute the first ever use of either randomization or a control group in science. The psychologist C. S. Peirce introduced the idea of randomization into his experiments in the 1880s (Stigler, 1986); and the American educationalists Thorndike and Woodworth used a control group in their experiments on the use of training to improve mental function in 1901 (Thorndike and Woodworth, 1901). The revolution for medical science was to use the two ideas together in the same experiment.

8. Syndromic STD management is based on the principle that certain symptoms—which collectively constitute a "syndrome"—are generally associated with a particular group of organisms. For example, urethral discharge is a syndrome that is usually caused by either gonorrhea or chlamydia. When it is not feasible to identify which pathogen is causing the condition, as in many rural African settings, the syndromic management approach would involve treating both. Acting thus, it is relatively certain that the agent responsible will be eliminated.

Chapter 3

1. In August 1972, President Amin declared what he called the Economic War, in which he expelled the 80,000 Asians living in Uganda, and set about expropriating their properties.

2. Hooper presents convincing evidence of a link between the route taken by the Tanzanian army's 207th Battalion during the war, and subsequent very high rates of AIDS in particular parts of Rakai and Masaka.

3. The word "charming" refers to witchcraft.

4. A longitudinal cohort study conducted from 1990 onwards by the Medical Research Council in rural Masaka found that the median period between HIV infection and death was 9.8 years (Morgan et al., 2002). However, the dynamics of an infection recently introduced into a population are different from the dynamics of one that is well established (Lipsitch and Nowak, 1995). Pathogens can be much more virulent early on in an epidemic, which explains why, during the early 1980s, many people died from AIDS so soon after being infected.

5. *Mukene* are small fish, up to eight centimeters long or so, that are caught in Lake Victoria and then dried. They are widely eaten locally.

6. Fishing settlements along the lakeshore are known as landing sites. They attract women who sell sex, and they tend to have very high HIV prevalence rates.

7. Elections in December 1980 returned Milton Obote to power. The subsequent conflict between the Ugandan army and Yoweri Museveni's insurgent National Resistance Army resulted in extensive violence and human rights abuses in many parts of the country.

8. Before the AIDS epidemic, African Kaposi's sarcoma was responsible for 9 percent of all cancers affecting Ugandan males (Taylor et al., 1971), and it was endemic in the areas of the Congo River and Lake Victoria basins. It generally presented peripherally (i.e., on the limbs and other extremities), and it was usually amenable to treatment.

9. Between 1982 and 1986, a bitter debate raged over the name and identity of the causative agent of AIDS. Luc Montagnier's lab at the Pasteur Institute in Paris isolated what he believed to be the agent, and called it LAV (Lymphadenopathy Associated Virus), while Robert Gallo's lab at the National Cancer Institute in Bethesda, Maryland, had called his isolate HTLV-III (Human T-cell Lymphotrophic Virus type 3). They were eventually shown to be the same virus, which in May 1986 was renamed HIV (Human Immunodeficiency Virus) by an international commission on virological nomenclature. See Grmek (1990) for further discussion.

10. There had been a few previous reports of African AIDS patients—from Zaire, Chad, and Mali—presenting in European hospitals (Offenstadt et al., 1983; Vittecoq and Modai, 1983; Clumeck et al., 1985), and one of a Ugandan woman who had died in London in 1983 (Edwards et al., 1984). No cases had yet been reported of African AIDS cases *in Africa*.

11. Robert Gallo was the American virologist who, in April 1984, named the virus that causes AIDS HTLV-III (see also Chapter 3, note 9).

12. Unfortunately, I was unable to meet with either Dr. M or Professor B to ask for their recollection of events, or for the rationale behind their thinking at the time, so I felt it necessary to protect their anonymity by giving them pseudonyms.

13. Other members of the team included Bob Downing, David Serwadda, Nelson Sewankambo, and Roy Mugerwa.

14. With regard to the ethics of this and his subsequent AIDS research, Carswell explained that "in all people from whom we took blood, we said that we were

testing for Slim which was widely known as a very serious condition. A few people declined." Carswell and his colleagues did not, however, have official permission to conduct the work. As he said, "this was a time of no effective administration. The Ethics Committee had not even met for about eight years." Nonetheless, they did inform the authorities of their findings: "Over the critical 18-month period in which most of the initial HTLV-III work was carried out, there were three consecutive administrations. I personally spoke to each of the three succeeding Ministers of Health to keep them informed of the HTLV-III/AIDS situation. Each gave implicit consent to the work that I carried out."

15. Data had been collected on four HTLV-III-related KS patients in the Uganda Cancer Institute at Mulago hospital between October 1983 and December 1984 (Serwadda et al., 1986). However, this study was not published until April 1986.

16. "Obote 2" is the name often given to Milton Obote's second presidency, from 1980 to 1985, during which an estimated 300,000 people were killed during the "war in the bush" between the Ugandan army and Yoweri Museveni's National Resistance Army. Obote was overthrown by Tito Okello in July 1985, who ruled over the warring nation for just six months before Museveni took power in January 1986.

17. These tests had worked by mixing blood with antibodies to HTLV-III, and if the virus itself was also present in the blood, then the virus and antibodies would combine to form a complex that would stick together. This could be seen, and would identify the sample as positive for HTLV-III. The problem was that the blood of people who were simultaneously parasitically infected—for example, with malaria—produced sticky complexes that were indistinguishable from complexes formed by HTLV-III; and since many people in rural Africa have malaria parasites in their blood, the result was a very large proportion of false HTLV-III-positive readings (Garrett, 1994:356).

18. Annual AIDS incidence rates were estimated in both studies by taking the number of AIDS cases presenting at the hospital during the investigation, assuming a similar rate for a 12-month period, and then extrapolating the 12-month estimate to the city's total population (Kinshasa or Kigali). Given that many AIDS patients would not have made it to the hospital, both estimates were therefore low.

19. "S" was an official at the Ministry of Health.

Chapter 4

1. There are of course also the higher-level issues, such as gender and economic inequalities, that can lead people into risky situations, but these are not especially amenable to an individual-level intervention approach. While these issues are clearly of great significance, they are not, however, the primary focus of this chapter.

2. The word "partners" refers here to people living in polygamous relationships, a fairly common practice in Uganda, and especially so within the Muslim community.
3. Distribution of female condoms did not begin in Uganda until 1997, when just 3,600 were sold—as compared to over 16 million male condoms that same year (DKT International, 2006).
4. Democratically elected Resistance Councils (RCs) had been established by Museveni, from village level all the way up to district level. RCs were responsible for overseeing service provision of all types in their respective areas.
5. Bishop Ddungu explained that he occasionally made *ad limina* visits—or pilgrimages—to Rome to see the tombs of the Apostles, the Pope, and the four basilicas. Church business was also conducted during these visits.
6. Longitudinal epidemiological cohort studies involve following up a number of individuals in a specified population over a period of time.
7. MRC and Rakai Project research during the early 1990s consisted primarily of descriptive epidemiological work, with the two organizations' social science departments also focusing on issues to do with stigma, marital instability, counseling, trust in condoms, and social support for people living with AIDS.
8. *Mzungu* is Swahili for "white person," and is a widely used term in Uganda. *Bazungu* is the plural.
9. TASO = The AIDS Support Organisation.
10. Observational evidence had emerged showing that HIV prevalence was lower in some populations among men who were circumcised—such as Muslims—as compared to their uncircumcised peers (Wagner et al., 1992). Circumcision was not definitively shown to be protective against HIV, however, until a series of three experimental studies—in South Africa, Uganda, and Kenya—were completed in 2007 (Auvert et al., 2005; Gray et al., 2007; Bailey et al., 2007).
11. Social marketing was established as a discipline in the early 1970s, with the recognition that the same marketing principles that are used to sell products to consumers could also be used to sell ideas, attitudes, and behaviors (Kotler and Zaltman, 1971). Social marketing was seen as a planned approach to social change, through the design and implementation of programs aimed at improving the acceptability and uptake of ideas and products.
12. See note 8 above.
13. Life Guard condoms made their debut in Uganda in 1996, with support from Marie Stopes International, a large NGO focusing on sexual and reproductive health issues.
14. The MRC's MIT is the topic of Chapter 6.
15. STI = Sexually Transmitted Infection.
16. In 1995, 48 percent of Ugandans were aged 15 or more, and the average age of first sex was 16.0 for women and 17.6 for men (DHS, 1996:9, 78).
17. Most epidemiological HIV surveillance relies on convenience samples, such as pregnant women attending antenatal clinics. While these are invaluable for establishing epidemiological trends, they are biased—not representative of the general population—so it is difficult to estimate overall HIV prevalence rates.

By contrast, general population cohorts are made up of all the adults living in a given geographical area who are willing to take part in ongoing, longitudinal surveillance, and as such they are far more representative. They are also, however, expensive and technically complex to manage. The general population cohorts in Masaka and Rakai were at this stage the only ones studying AIDS in all of Africa.

18. The United States Leadership Against HIV/AIDS, Tuberculosis, and Malaria Act of 2003.

19. VCT = Voluntary HIV Counseling and Testing.

20. *Engabo* means "shield" in Museveni's mother tongue, Runyankore.

Chapter 5

1. See Whyte (1992) for a detailed discussion of the nature of the professional and folk health care sectors in rural Eastern Uganda.

2. The three most commonly used classes of ARVs are (i) nucleoside reverse transcriptase inhibitors (NRTIs), (ii) non-nucleoside reverse transcriptase inhibitors (NNR-TIs), and (iii) protease inhibitors. They all work by inhibiting the activities of particular enzymes that are necessary for viral replication.

3. Around 930,000 Ugandans were estimated to be living with HIV in 1997 (UNAIDS, 1998:65), of whom somewhere between 10 percent and 20 percent (93,000 to 186,000 people) would have been severely immunosuppressed and therefore clinically eligible for ART.

4. These included (i) antibiotics for treating STDs, (ii) drugs for OIs, and (iii) ARVs.

5. NDA = National Drug Authority.

6. IAS = International AIDS Society.

7. See, for example, Dukers et al. (2001) for a description of this phenomenon in Amsterdam.

8. While extended life inevitably brings about "additional opportunities" for transmission, it is important to note that since ART reduces viral load, it also reduces an individual's infectiousness *per partner exposure*. Thus an HIV-positive person who is taking ART is very unlikely to transmit HIV in any given sex act. The argument here, however, suggests that their extended life may well include a large number of these lower-risk sex acts, thus making them more likely overall to transmit HIV. By contrast, had they died swiftly of AIDS and in the absence of ART, they would have been quite infectious per putative sex act, but they would doubtless also have been feeling quite poorly, and thus would likely have remained relatively celibate. In addition, their period of elevated infectiousness (i.e., before their premature death) would have been short. Thus they would have been unlikely overall to transmit the virus at this late stage of their illness.

9. In May 2007, President Bush announced U.S. plans to spend a further $30 billion over five years in Africa and elsewhere to combat HIV and AIDS. The subsequent legislation—the Tom Lantos and Henry J. Hyde United States Global

Leadership Against HIV/AIDS, Tuberculosis, and Malaria Reauthorization Act of 2008—actually authorized up to $48 billion for the period 2009 to 2013.

10. It is important to note that use of the term "Big Men" here does not in any way suggest that women have played no role in ART scale-up. However, apart from former WHO Director General Dr. Gro Harlem Bruntland (who first touted the idea of '3 by 5'), there have in fact been remarkably few women involved in the process at the most senior levels. This is mainly because the worlds of politics and finance tend to be male-dominated, and is not in any way an indication that women have not also been engaged and involved in the issue. Within the advocacy sphere, for example, women such as Ellen 't Hoen (formerly of MSF, and now leading UNITAID's efforts to launch an HIV patent pool that will keep down the cost of ARVs) have made a very significant impact.

11. DG = WHO Director General.

12. Dr. Yusuf Hamied is Chairman of Cipla, the Indian drug company that pioneered the production of cheap, generic ARVs.

13. CD4 cell counts are used as markers for determining a patient's level of immunosuppression. Most healthy people have around 1,000 CD4 cells/mm^3; WHO's 2002 guidelines recommended that ART be initiated when the CD4 count drops to 200 (WHO, 2002b), by when people have often started to fall sick with AIDS-related diseases. Current guidelines call for earlier initiation of therapy, when the CD4 count reaches 350 (WHO, 2009b).

14. The various ARV providers in Uganda in late 2004 included the Ministry of Health; JCRC; various NGOs such as MSF, GTZ, TASO, and Mildmay; the Uganda Business Coalition and Uganda Cares; private-for-profit providers; and a number of research programs.

15. In the early-mid 1990s, David Ho's research focus was the dynamic nature of HIV replication in infected people, which contributed to his groundbreaking work in the development of one of the three main classes of ARVs, protease inhibitors. He was named *Time* magazine's Man of the Year in 1996.

16. The other co-organizers included the Community Health and Information Network (CHAIN), the Ugandan Business Coalition on HIV/AIDS, and the Ugandan Ministry of Health.

17. This is by no means to suggest that all public health scientists opposed rapid ART scale-up—there are many issues in international public health on which there is no collectively agreed view. Indeed, as explained above, it was public health and clinical scientists who provided the evidence from small-scale pilot projects that was then used to justify the arguments of the activists, politicians, and financiers pushing for scale-up.

Chapter 6

1. Garrett (1994:355–359) describes how Western scientists at this time would fly into African countries, take samples from AIDS patients—frequently without adequate informed consent procedures or ethical clearance—and then fly

home with the samples, only to publish their findings without any national coauthors, and without any attempt to obtain comments or clearance from the appropriate authorities.

2. This was an astonishingly prescient estimate. The UNAIDS report for 2000 estimated that 24.5 million Africans were living with HIV in that year—as opposed to the 25 million that had been predicted eight years earlier (UNAIDS, 2000).

3. As described in Chapter 4, the MRC's Kyamulibwa cohort had been established in order to provide an understanding of changing HIV infection and associated mortality rates, as well as of sexual behavior patterns in rural Masaka.

4. Studies in neighboring Zaire had shown some STDs to act as powerful cofactors for HIV infection. For example, the presence of gonorrhea increased the chance of HIV sero-conversion by 4.8 times, while chlamydia increased the chance by 3.6 times (Laga et al., 1993; see also Wasserheit, 1992). It was therefore hypothesized that treating such STDs could act as a means of HIV prevention.

   More recently, convincing evidence has emerged that male circumcision can be protective against HIV infection (Auvert et al., 2005; Gray et al., 2007; Bailey et al., 2007); and ARVs are now widely used in the prevention of mother-to-child HIV transmission. Universal voluntary HIV testing with immediate antiretroviral therapy has also been proposed as a strategy for the elimination of HIV transmission (Granich et al., 2009).

5. See Chapter 2, note 8, for an explanation of syndromic STD management.

6. The key players in the Mwanza team and the MRC Programme on AIDS in Uganda were all closely connected to the London School of Hygiene and Tropical Medicine, and were all well acquainted with each other.

7. A Ugandan Parish is an official administrative unit, comprised of between 5 and 15 villages.

8. Treatment algorithms are standardized guidelines used by clinicians for treating specific conditions and syndromes.

9. A community randomized trial is a form of randomized controlled trial (as defined and discussed in Chapter 2), in which communities—rather than individuals—are randomly assigned to either the intervention or the control group.

10. As per internationally accepted ethical standards, informed consent was required from all study participants, and nobody was obliged to take part.

11. WHO/GPA, UNAIDS, and MRC all funded the MIT to different degrees at different points in its life.

12. MIT paid staff included a project leader, five people working on IEC, two on STDs, two on community development, a large survey team, four data entry officers, a laboratory technician, several drivers, two administrative staff, and two security staff with a dog to protect the office and compound.

13. Longitudinal (or follow-up) data had been collected from 13,500 people—meaning that they had been surveyed and bled more than once, and could therefore contribute to the calculations on HIV and STD incidence. A further 7,000 or so had been seen just once, which meant that they could not contribute to these calculations, but they could still provide demographic and other data.

14. ABC = Abstinence, Be faithful, and use Condoms. See Chapter 4 for detailed discussion.

15. Costs were estimated in 2001 dollars, and included only the implementation of the intervention. Research costs—such as serological tests, as well as salaries and transport for scientific staff and the survey team—were not included in this figure.

16. It is also worth mentioning that a further analysis of the MIT dataset—at individual level rather than community level, an important epidemiological distinction—showed that there had in fact been a significant reduction in HIV incidence, specifically among women who had attended the intervention activities (Quigley et al., 2004). However, the impact of these findings, which add yet another layer of complexity to the issue, was substantially less than that of the initial paper. A Google Scholar search of Quigley et al. (2004) in December 2009 found that it had been cited in just 20 other scientific papers, as compared to the main MIT paper (Kamali et al., 2003), which had been cited 165 times.

17. This consensus was derived through epidemiological analysis of the three study populations, which showed that there was (i) more high-risk behavior and (ii) higher rates of bacterial—and therefore treatable—STDs in Mwanza than in the two Ugandan cohorts. Thus there was more room for reducing incidence rates in Mwanza, and inherently, therefore, a greater chance of a positive result (Rutherford, 2002:85).

18. This hypothesis was subsequently rebuffed in a *Lancet* article that argued that "although there is a clear need to eliminate all unsafe injections, epidemiological evidence indicates that sexual transmission continues to be by far the major mode of spread of HIV-1 in the region. Increased efforts are needed to reduce sexual transmission of HIV-1" (Schmid et al., 2004:482).

19. Volunteers were given up to 10,000 Uganda shillings—around $6—for one day's assistance in guiding the survey team to particular households in the study parish.

20. The respondent is referring to paid MRC staff.

21. The bleeder was a member of the survey team who took blood samples from study participants.

22. A *panga* is a long-bladed machete widely used in Ugandan agricultural work.

23. Many people in the villages can not read or write.

24. Given the difficulties that would certainly have been faced at these meetings if the full epidemiological picture from the trial had been given, MRC staff only provided village-level HIV prevalence data obtained during the three survey rounds. Since there had been a fall in prevalence throughout the study area, this could easily have been interpreted in most villages as indicating intervention success.

Chapter 7

1. One important exception to this was a groundbreaking RCT conducted between 1997 and 1999 in Kampala to evaluate the effectiveness of an ARV,

nevirapine, as a means of reducing mother-to-child transmission of HIV. The study showed that nevirapine could lower the risk of transmission during the first 14–16 weeks of life by nearly 50 percent in a breastfeeding population (Guay et al., 1999), and it had a significant impact on policy for preventing mother-to-child transmission. This particular arena of AIDS control has, however, fallen outside the remit of this book.

2. One observer has written of the "complexity of the field and the degree of disagreement within it; nobody has yet come up with a single comprehensive definition of ideology acceptable to all concerned" (Eagleton, 1994:20).

3. Pragmatism in philosophy is a principle of enquiry first put forward by Charles Sanders Peirce in the 1870s, and which acted as a forerunner to logical positivism.

References

Abdool Karim S., J. Currier, C. del Rio, J. Feinberg, G. Friedland, P. Sax, A. Zuger. 2002. Report on the Fourteenth International AIDS Conference. *AIDS Clinical Care* 14(9): 77–85.

ACP. 1989a. *Progress on the AIDS epidemic in Uganda, 1987–89.* Entebbe: AIDS Control Programme, Ministry of Health.

———. 1989b. *AIDS surveillance report, fourth quarter 1989.* Entebbe: AIDS Control Programme, Ministry of Health.

———. 1990. *AIDS surveillance report, third quarter 1990.* Entebbe: AIDS Control Programme, Ministry of Health.

———. 1991. *AIDS surveillance report, first and second quarters 1991.* Entebbe: AIDS Control Programme, Ministry of Health.

———. 1992. *AIDS surveillance report, June 1992.* Entebbe: AIDS Control Programme, Ministry of Health.

———. 1999. *HIV/AIDS surveillance report.* Entebbe: AIDS Control Programme, Ministry of Health.

———. 2000. *HIV/AIDS surveillance report, June 2000.* Kampala: STD/AIDS Control Programme, Ministry of Health.

———. 2003. *National condom policy and strategy—draft, June 2003.* Kampala: STD/AIDS Control Programme.

———. 2004. *National condom policy and strategy.* Kampala: STD/AIDS Control Programme, Ministry of Health.

Adams J., and M. Hillman. 2001. The risk compensation theory and bicycle helmets. *Injury Prevention* 7:89–91.

Adler E., and P. Haas. 1992. Epistemic communities, world order, and the creation of a reflective research program. *International Organization* 46(1): 367–390.

AHF. 2005. *AIDS Healthcare Foundation, Consolidated Financial Statements and Supplementary Information, Dec 31, 2004 and 2003.* http://www.aidshealth.org/assets/pdf/2005-2004.pdf. Accessed November 21, 2009.

———. 2009. *AHF in Uganda.* http://www.aidshealth.org/assets/pdf/country-reports/uganda-fact-sheet.pdf. Accessed December 8, 2009.

AIDS Analysis Africa. 1992. AIDS and behaviour change: A statement of belief. *AIDS Analysis Africa, Southern Africa Edition* 3(1): 6.

Altman D. 1998. Globalization and the "AIDS industry." *Contemporary Politics* 4(3): 233–245.

Anderson J. 1989. Uganda's pioneering support organisation. *AIDS Watch* (6): 8.

Ankrah M. 1989. AIDS: Methodological problems in studying its prevention and spread. *Social Science and Medicine* 29(3): 265–276.

Arnold J. 2000. *History: A very short introduction.* Oxford: Oxford University Press.

Asamoah-Adu A., S. Weir, M. Pappoe, N. Kanlisi, A. Neequaye, P. Lamptey. 1994. Evaluation of a targeted AIDS prevention intervention to increase condom use among prostitutes in Ghana. *AIDS* 8(2): 239–246.

Auvert B., D. Taljaard, E. Lagarde, J. Sobngwi-Tambekou, R. Sitta, A. Puren. 2005. Randomized, controlled intervention trial of male circumcision for reduction of HIV infection risk: The ANRS 1265 trial. *Public Library of Science Medicine* 2(11): e298. doi:10.1371/journal.pmed.0020298.

Avert. 2006. *PEPFAR: How is the money to be divided between different areas of work?* http://www.avert.org/pepfar.htm. Accessed November 23, 2009.

Bachengana C. 1995. *A situational analysis of sex education in schools.* Presentation, Ninth International Conference on AIDS and STD in Africa, Kampala.

Baer H., M. Singer, J. Johnsen. 1986. Toward a critical medical anthropology. *Social Science and Medicine* 23(2): 95–98.

Bailey R., S. Moses, C. Parker. 2007. Male circumcision for HIV prevention in young men in Kisumu, Kenya: A randomised controlled trial. *Lancet* 369:643–656.

Barnett T., and P. Blaikie. 1992. *AIDS in Africa—Its present and future impact.* New York: Guilford Press.

Basajja V., A. Kamali, J. Kinsman, J. Whitworth. 2000. *A community-based condom social marketing strategy in rural Uganda.* Oral Presentation MoOrC244, Thirteenth International AIDS Conference, Durban.

Bass E. 2005. Fighting to close the condom gap in Uganda. *Lancet* 365(9465): 1127–1128.

Bayley A. 1984. Aggressive Kaposi's sarcoma in Zambia, 1983. *Lancet* 323(8390): 1318–1320.

Bayley A., R. Downing, R. Cheingsong-Popov, R. Tedder, A. Dalgleish, R. Weiss. 1985. HTLV-III serology distinguishes atypical and endemic Kaposi's sarcoma in Africa. *Lancet* 325(8425): 359–361.

Bessinger R., P. Akwara, D. Halperin. 2003. *Sexual behavior, HIV and fertility trends: A comparative analysis of six countries; phase I of the ABC study.* Chapel Hill, NC: Measure Evaluation.

Beuving J. 2006. *Cotonou's Klondike: A sociological analysis of entrepreneurship in the Euro-West African second-hand car trade.* Enschede, the Netherlands: Febo Press.

Bijker W., and J. Law. 1992. *Shaping technology/building society: Studies in sociotechnical change.* Cambridge, MA: MIT Press.

Black N. 2001. Evidence based policy: Proceed with care. *British Medical Journal* 323:275–279.

Bonell C. 2002. The politics of the research-policy interface: Randomised trials and the commissioning of HIV prevention services. *Sociology of Health and Illness* 24(4): 385–408.

Boston Globe. 2003. HIV rate may be declining in Africa. Boston, MA, May 11.

Bourdieu P. 1977. *Outline of a theory of practice.* Cambridge: Cambridge University Press.

———. 1992. *The Logic of Practice.* Stanford: Stanford University Press.

———. 1999. *Pascalian meditations.* Cambridge: Polity.

Bowen S., and A. Zwi. 2005. Pathways to "evidence-informed" policy and practice: A framework for action. *Public Library of Science Medicine* 2(7): e166. doi:10.1371/journal.pmed.0020166.

Brunt L., and H. Ronden. 1991. The enemy without a face: Cholera in Amsterdam, 1832. In *Economic and Social History in the Netherlands, Volume III*, pp 81–98. Amsterdam: Netherlands Economic History Archive.

Bush G. 2003a. President delivers "State of the Union." http://georgewbush-whitehouse.archives.gov/news/releases/2003/01/20030128-19.html. Accessed November 25, 2009.

———. 2003b. President signs HIV/AIDS Act. http://georgewbush-whitehouse.archives.gov/news/releases/2003/05/20030527-7.html. Accessed November 25, 2009.

Buvé A., E. Lagarde, M. Caraël, N. Rutenberg, B. Ferry, J. R. Glynn, M. Laourou, E. Akam, J. Chege, T. Sukwa. 2001. Interpreting sexual behaviour data: Validity issues in the multicentre study on factors determining the differential spread of HIV in four African cities. *AIDS* 15(S4): S117–S126.

Campbell C. 2003. *Letting them die: Why HIV/AIDS prevention programmes fail.* Oxford: James Currey.

Carswell W. 1987. HIV infection in healthy persons in Uganda. *AIDS* 1(4): 223–227.

Cassell M., D. Halperin, J. Shelton, D. Stanton. 2006. Risk compensation: The Achilles' heel of innovations in HIV prevention? *British Medical Journal* 332:605–607.

Catholic Bishops of Uganda. 1989. *The AIDS epidemic—Message of the Catholic Bishops of Uganda.* Kampala: Marianum Press.

Catholic Hierarchy. 2006. *Diocese of Masaka, statistics.* www.catholic-hierarchy.org/diocese/dmska.html. Accessed November 24, 2009.

CDC. 1981. Pneumocystis pneumonia—Los Angeles. *Morbidity and Mortality Weekly Report* 30(21): 250–252.

Clifford J., and G. Marcus. 1986. *Writing culture: The poetics and politics of ethnography.* Berkeley: University of California Press.

Clumeck N., M. Robert-Guroff, P. Van de Perre, A. Jennings, J. Sibomana, P. Demol, S. Cran, R. Gallo. 1985. Seroepidemiological studies of HTLV-III antibody prevalence among selected groups of heterosexual Africans. *Journal of the American Medical Association* 254(18): 2599–2602.

Cochrane. 2006. *The Cochrane collaboration.* www.cochrane.org. Accessed November 24, 2009.

Cohen S. 2004. Beyond slogans: Lessons from Uganda's experience with ABC and HIV/AIDS. *Reproductive Health Matters* 12(23): 132–135.

Court J. 2004. *Bridging research and policy on HIV/AIDS in developing countries.* London: Overseas Development Institute.

Court J., and S. Maxwell. 2005. Policy entrepreneurship for poverty reduction: Bridging research and policy in international development. *Journal of International Development* 17(6): 713–725.

Cushman C. 2005. Burying their hope. *Citizen*, April:18–25. http://www.citizenlink. org/citizenmag/. Accessed November 24, 2009.

Dare O., and J. Cleland. 1994. Reliability and validity of survey data on sexual behaviour. *Health Transition Review* 4 (Supplement): 93–110.

Davies H., and S. Nutley. 2002. *Evidence-based policy and practice: Moving from rhetoric to reality.* February 2002. Discussion Paper. University of St. Andrews, Research Unit for Research Utilisation.

Debrow M., V. Goel, R. Upshur. 2004. Evidence-based health policy: Context and utilization. *Social Science and Medicine* 58(1): 207–217.

Dehue T. 2004. Historiography taking issue: Analyzing an experiment with heroin abusers. *Journal of the History of the Behavioral Sciences* 40(3): 247–264.

Demers A., S. Kairouz, E. Adlaf, L. Gliksman, B. Newton-Taylor, A. Marchand. 2002. Multilevel analysis of situational drinking among Canadian undergraduates. *Social Science and Medicine* 55(3): 415–424.

DHS. 1996. *Uganda Demographic and Health Survey, 1995.* Entebbe: Ministry of Finance and Economic Planning, Statistics Department; Calverton, MD: Macro International Inc., Demographic and Health Surveys.

Diez-Roux A. 2000. Multilevel analysis in public health research. *Annual Review of Public Health* 21: 171–192.

DKT International. 2006. *Uganda social marketing program.*

Dobson J. 2003. Dobson calls for quick Senate action on global AIDS Bill. May 14. http://www.charitywire.com/charity63/03878.html. Accessed November 24, 2009.

Donald A. 2001. Research must be taken seriously. *British Medical Journal* 323: 278–279.

Duesberg P. 1997. *Inventing the AIDS virus.* Washington, D.C.: Regnery Publishing.

Dukers N., J. Goudsmit, J. de Wit, M. Prins, G. Weverling, R. Coutinho. 2001. Sexual risk behaviour relates to the virological and immunological improvements during highly active antiretroviral therapy in HIV-1 infection. *AIDS* 15(3): 369–378.

Duncan C., K. Jones, G. Moon. 1998. Context, composition and heterogeneity: Using multilevel models in health research. *Social Science and Medicine* 46(1): 97–117.

Durban Declaration. 2000. *Nature* 406:15–16.

Eagleton T. 1994. *Ideology.* London: Longman.

———. 2007. *Ideology—An introduction.* London: Verso.

East African. 2005. Uganda surpasses target of people on ARVs by 11 percent. Nairobi, December 6.

Edwards D., P. Harper, A. Pain, J. Welch, C. Barbatis, C. Mallinson. 1984. Kaposi's sarcoma associated with AIDS in a woman from Uganda. *Lancet* 323(8377): 631–632.

Epstein H. 2007. *The invisible cure: Africa, the West and the fight against AIDS.* London: Viking.

Evans M., and J. Davies. 1999. Understanding policy transfer: A multi-level, multi-disciplinary perspective. *Public Administration* 77(2): 361–385.

Evans R. 1995. Epidemics and revolutions: Cholera in nineteenth century Europe. In *Epidemics and ideas: Essays on the historical perception of pestilence,* ed. T. Ranger and P. Slack, pp 149–174. Cambridge: Cambridge University Press.

Evidence-Based Medicine Working Group. 1992. A new approach to teaching the practice of medicine. *Journal of the American Medical Association* 268: 2420–2425.

Farmer P. 1993. *AIDS and accusation: Haiti and the geography of blame.* Berkeley: University of California Press.

———. 2001. *Infections and inequalities: The modern plagues.* Berkeley: University of California Press.

Ferriman A. 2001. UN calls for $10bn to wage war on AIDS. *British Medical Journal* 322(7294): 1082.

Fischer D. 1970. *Historians' fallacies: Toward a logic of historical thought.* New York: Harper Collins.

Fleming D., and J. Wasserheit. 1999. From epidemiological synergy to public health policy and practice: The contribution of other sexually transmitted diseases to sexual transmission of HIV infection. *Sexually Transmitted Infections* 75(1): 3–17.

Fountain. 1992. *Uganda—30 years.* Kampala: Fountain Publishers Ltd.

Fuchs F., M. Klag, P. Whelton. 2000. The classics: A tribute to the fiftieth anniversary of the randomized clinical trial. *Journal of Clinical Epidemiology* 53(4): 335–342.

Furay C., and M. Salevouris. 1988. *The methods and skills of history: A practical guide.* Wheeling, IL: Harlan Davidson.

G8. 2005. *Africa communiqué.* http://data.unaids.org/Topics/UniversalAccess/PostG8_Gleneagles_Africa_en.pdf. Accessed December 9, 2009.

Garner P., M. Meremikwu, J. Volmink, Q. Xu, H. Smith. 2004. Putting evidence into practice: How middle and low income countries "get it together." *British Medical Journal* 329: 1036–1039.

Garnett G. 2003. *Combined strategies for successful HIV control.* Keynote address, Fifteenth International Society for STD Research conference, Ottawa.

Garrett L. 1994. *The coming plague.* London: Virago.

Gayle H., and J. Lange. 2004. Seizing the opportunity to capitalise on the growing access to HIV treatment to expand HIV prevention. *Lancet* 364(9428): 6–8.

Gisselquist D., J. Potterat, S. Brody, F. Vachon. 2003. Let it be sexual: How health care transmission of AIDS in Africa was ignored. *International Journal of STD and AIDS* 14(3): 148–161.

Global Fund. 2003. Global Fund signs US$36.3 million grant to support Uganda's ongoing fight against HIV/AIDS. Geneva. http://www.theglobalfund.org/en/pressreleases/?pr=pr_030227b. Accessed November 24, 2009.

Goodrich J., K. Wellings, D. McVey. 1998. Using condom data to assess the impact of HIV/AIDS preventive interventions. *Health Education Research* 13(2): 267–274.

GRADE Working Group. 2004. Grading quality of evidence and strength of recommendations. *British Medical Journal* 328:1490–1497.

Granich R., C. Gilks, C. Dye, K. de Cock, B. Williams. 2009. Universal voluntary HIV testing with immediate antiretroviral therapy as a strategy for elimination of HIV transmission: A mathematical model. *Lancet* 373:48–57.

Gray R., G. Kigozi, D. Serwadda, F. Makumbi, S. Watya, F. Nalugoda, N. Kiwanuka, et al. 2007. Male circumcision for HIV prevention in men in Rakai, Uganda: A randomised trial. *Lancet* 369(9562): 657–666.

Gray R., M. Wawer, R. Brookmeyer, N. Sewankambo, D. Serwadda, F. Wabwire-Mangen, F. Lutalo, X. Li, T. vanCott, T. Quinn. 2001. Probability of HIV-1 transmission per coital act in monogamous heterosexual, HIV-1 discordant couples in Rakai, Uganda. *Lancet* 357(9263): 1149–1153.

Green E. 2003a. Testimony before the African subcommittee U.S. Senate, May 19, 2003. http://www.kaisernetwork.org/health_cast/hcast_index.cfm?create=high_windows&linkid=1&display=detail&hc=873. Accessed November 24, 2009.

———. 2003b. *Rethinking AIDS prevention: Learning from success in developing countries.* Westport, CT; London: Praeger.

———. 2004. AIDS debate in Anthropology News—A synopsis and final comments. *Anthropology News*, January.

Grmek M. 1990. *History of AIDS: Emergence and origin of a modern epidemic.* Princeton, NJ: Princeton University Press.

Grosskurth H., F. Mosha, J. Todd, E. Mwijarubi, A. Klokke, K. Senkoro, P. Mayaud, J. Changalucha, A. Nicoll, G. ka-Gina. 1995. Impact of improved treatment of sexually transmitted diseases on HIV infection in Tanzania: Randomised controlled trial. *Lancet* 346(8974): 530–536.

Grosskurth H., R. Gray, R. Hayes, D. Mabey, M. Wawer. 2000. Control of sexually transmitted diseases for HIV-1 prevention: Understanding the implications of the Mwanza and Rakai trials. *Lancet* 355(9219): 1981–1987.

Guardian. 2001. Crusading Indian firm takes on might of GlaxoSmithKline. February 14. London.

———. 2002. Aids drugs bring hope to South Africa. January 30. London.

———. 2003. Ruling opens the door for cut-price HIV drugs. October 17. London.

Guay L., P. Musoke, T. Fleming, D. Bagenda, M. Allen, C. Nakabiito, J. Sherman, et al. 1999. Intrapartum and neonatal single-dose nevirapine compared with zidovudine for prevention of mother-to-child transmission of HIV-1 in Kampala, Uganda: HIVNET 012 randomised trial. *Lancet* 354(9181): 795–802.

Halperin D., M. Steiner, M. Cassell, E. Green, N. Hearst, D. Kirby, H. Gayle, W. Cates. 2004. The time has come for common ground on preventing sexual transmission of HIV. *Lancet* 364(9449): 1913–1915.

Haraway D. 1991. *Simians, cyborgs and women: The reinvention of nature.* London: Free Association Books.

Hardon A., D. Akurut, C. Comoro, C. Ekezie, H. Irunde, T. Gerrits, J. Kgatlwane, et al. 2007. Hunger, waiting time and transport costs: Time to confront challenges to ART adherence in Africa. *AIDS Care* 19(5): 658–665.

Hardon A., P. Boonmongkon, P. Streefland, M. Tan, T. Hongvivatana, S. van der Geest, A. van Staa, et al. 1994. *Applied health research: Anthropology of health and health care.* Amsterdam: Het Spinhuis.

Harries A., D. Nyangulu, N. Hargreaves, O. Kaluwa, F. Salaniponi. 2001. Preventing antiretroviral anarchy in sub-Saharan Africa. *Lancet* 358(9279): 410–414.

Hayes R., F. Mosha, A. Nicoll, H. Grosskurth, J. Newell, J. Todd, J. Killewo, J. Rugemalila, D. Mabey. 1995. A community trial of the impact of improved sexually transmitted disease treatment on the HIV epidemic in rural Tanzania: 1. Design. *AIDS* 9(8): 919–926.

Health Evidence Network. 2006. *Health evidence network, homepage.* http://www.euro.who.int/HEN. Accessed November 24, 2009.

Heckert K., and M. Baldo. 1998. *Best practices in school AIDS/life skills education: Selected case studies.* Abstract 13499, Twelfth International AIDS Conference, Geneva.

Hennekens C., and J. Buring. 1987. *Epidemiology in medicine.* Boston: Little Brown and Company.

Hitchcock P., and L. Fransen. 1999. Preventing HIV infection: Lessons from Mwanza and Rakai. *Lancet* 353(9152): 513–515.

Hogan D., and J. Salomon. 2005. Prevention and treatment of human immunodeficiency virus/acquired immunodeficiency syndrome in resource-poor settings. *Bulletin of the World Health Organization* 83:135–143.

Hogle J., E. Green, V. Nantulya, R. Stoneburner, J. Stover. 2002. *What happened in Uganda? Declining HIV prevalence, behavior change, and the national response.* Washington, D.C.: USAID.

Hooper E. 1999. *The river.* Boston: Little, Brown and Company.

Horchler S., A. Gerhardus, G. Schmidt-Ehry, B. Schmidt-Ehry, R. Korte, S. Mitra, R. Sauerborn. 2004. The role of research in a technical assistance agency: The case of the German agency for technical co-operation. *Health Policy* 70: 229–241.

Hubley J. 2006. Leeds health education database; interventions to control AIDS and sexually transmitted diseases. http://www.hubley.co.uk/db-aids.htm#part12. Accessed November 24, 2009.

Human Rights Watch. 2005. The less they know, the better—Abstinence-only HIV/AIDS programs in Uganda. http://www.hrw.org/reports/2005/uganda0305/index.htm. Accessed November 24, 2009.

Hyde K., A. Ekatan, P. Kiage, C. Baraswa. 2002. *The impact of HIV/AIDS on formal schooling in Uganda.* New York: Rockefeller Foundation.

Iliffe J. 1998. *East African doctors—A history of the modern profession.* Kampala: Fountain Publishers.

Independent. 2000. African AIDS epidemic "could cause revolution and war." 1 May. London.

INFORMS. 2004. *O. R.: The science of better*. Hanover, MD: Institute for Operations Research and the Management Sciences. http://www.scienceofbetter.org/. Accessed December 12, 2009.

IPPPH. 2003. *Impact of public-private partnerships addressing access to pharmaceuticals in low income countries—Uganda pilot study*. Geneva: Initiative on Public-Private Partnerships for Health.

IRIN. 2002. Row over HIV/AIDS success story. August 23. http://www.plusnews.org/report.aspx?ReportId=31409. Accessed November 24, 2009.

———. 2006. Uganda: Condom shortage in north affecting HIV prevention efforts. http://www.irinnews.org/Report.aspx?ReportId=39693. Accessed November 24, 2009.

Jenkins R. 1992. *Pierre Bourdieu*. London: Routledge.

Jeppsson A., H. Birungi, P-O Östergren, B. Hagström. 2005. The global-local dilemma of a Ministry of Health—Experiences from Uganda. *Health Policy* 72:311–320.

Jones K., G. Moon, A. Clegg. 1991. Ecological and individual effects in childhood immunisation uptake: A multi-level approach. *Social Science and Medicine* 33(4): 501–508.

Justice J. 1987. The bureaucratic context of international health: A social scientist's view. *Social Science and Medicine* 25(12): 1301–1306.

Kager P. 1998. New epidemics: Possibilities for prevention and control. In *Problems and potential in international health: Transdisciplinary perspectives*, ed. P. Streefland, 11–35. Amsterdam: Het Spinhuis.

Kagimu M., E. Marum, F. Wabwire-Mangen, N. Nakyanjo, Y. Walakira, J. Hogle. 1998. Evaluation of the effectiveness of AIDS health education interventions in the Muslim community in Uganda. *AIDS Education and Prevention* 10(3): 215–228.

Kaiser Network. 2004. *Political commitment and accountability*. July 7, Fifteenth International AIDS Conference, Bangkok. http://www.kaisernetwork.org/health_cast/hcast_index.cfm?display=detail&hc=1189. Accessed November 24, 2009.

———. 2006. *Highlights from late breaker abstracts—Tracks B, C and D*. August 17, Sixteenth International AIDS Conference, Toronto. http://www.kaisernetwork.org/health_cast/hcast_index.cfm?display=detail&hc=1809#part2. Accessed November 24, 2009.

Kaleeba N., S. Kalibala, M. Kaseje, P. Ssebbanja, S. Anderson, E. van Praag, G. Tembo, E. Katabira. 1997. Participatory evaluation of counselling, medical and social services of The AIDS Support Organization (TASO) in Uganda. *AIDS Care* 9(1): 13–26.

Kaleeba N., S. Ray, B. Willmore. 1991. *We miss you all*. Harare, Zimbabwe: Women and AIDS Support Network (WASN).

Kalibala S., and N. Kaleeba. 1989. AIDS and community-based care in Uganda: The AIDS support organization, TASO. *AIDS Care* 1(2): 173–175.

Kamali A., J. Kinsman, N. Nalweyiso, K. Mitchell, E. Kanyesigye, J. Kengeya-Kayondo, L. Carpenter, A. Nunn, J. Whitworth. 2002. A community randomized controlled trial to investigate impact of improved STD management and behavioural interventions on HIV incidence in rural Masaka, Uganda: Trial design, methods and baseline findings. *Tropical Medicine and International Health* 7(12): 1053–1063.

Kamali A., L. Carpenter, J. Whitworth, R. Pool, A. Ruberantwari, A. Ojwiya. 2000. Seven-year trends in HIV-1 infection rates, and changes in sexual behaviour, among adults in rural Uganda. *AIDS* 14(4): 427–434.

Kamali A., M. Quigley, J. Nakiyingi, J. Kinsman, J. Kengeya-Kayondo, R. Gopal, A. Ojwiya, P. Hughes, L. Carpenter, J. Whitworth. 2003. Syndromic management of sexually-transmitted infections and behaviour change interventions on transmission of HIV-1 in rural Uganda: A community randomised trial. *Lancet* 361(9358): 645–652.

Kapiriri L., O. Norheim, K. Heggenhougen. 2003. Public participation in health planning and priority setting at the district level in Uganda. *Health Policy and Planning* 18(2): 205–213.

Kasper T., D. Coetzee, F. Louis, A. Boulle, K. Hilderbrand. 2003. Demystifying antiretroviral therapy in resource-poor settings. *Essential Drugs Monitor* (32): 20–21.

Katzenstein D., M. Laga, J. Moatti. 2003. The evaluation of the HIV/AIDS drug access initiatives in Côte D'Ivoire, Senegal and Uganda: How access to antiretroviral treatment can become feasible in Africa. *AIDS* 17(S3): S1–S4.

Kilian A., S. Gregson, B. Ndyanabangi, K. Walusaga, W. Kipp, G. Sahlmüller, G. Garnett, et al. 1999. Reductions in risk behaviour provide the most consistent explanation for declining HIV-1 prevalence in Uganda. *AIDS* 13(3): 391–398.

Kingdon J. 1984. *Agendas, alternatives and public policies.* Boston: Little Brown & Co.

Kinsman J., A. Kamali, E. Kanyesigye, I. Kamulegeya, V. Basajja, J. Nakiyingi, K. Schenk, J. Whitworth. 2002. Quantitative process evaluation of a community-based HIV/AIDS behavioural intervention in rural Uganda. *Health Education Research—Theory and Practice* 17(2): 253–265.

Kinsman J., I. Kamulegeya, K. Schenk, J. Nakiyingi, V. Basajja, A. Kamali, J. Whitworth. 2000. *Community-based AIDS education in rural Uganda—Can it work, and who should do it?* Oral Poster TuPpD1202, Thirteenth World AIDS Conference, Durban.

Kinsman J., J. Nakiyingi, A. Kamali, L. Carpenter, M. Quigley, R. Pool, J. Whitworth. 2001. Evaluation of a comprehensive school-based AIDS education programme in rural Masaka, Uganda. *Health Education Research—Theory and Practice* 16(1): 85–100.

Kinsman J., S. Harrison, J. Kengeya-Kayondo, E. Kanyesigye, S. Musoke, J. Whitworth. 1999. Implementation of a comprehensive school-based AIDS education programme in Masaka District, Uganda. *AIDS Care* 11(5): 591–601.

Kipp W., G. Kabagambe, J. Konde-Lule. 2001. Low impact of a community-wide HIV testing and counseling program on sexual behavior in rural Uganda. *AIDS Education and Prevention* 13(3): 279–289.

Kippax S. 2002. *Throwing the baby out with the bathwater: Unsuitability of experimental evaluations for sexual health interventions.* Abstract no. D11377, Fourteenth International AIDS Conference, Barcelona.

Kirumira E. 1992. Uganda: Why a re-think is needed of AIDS control policy. *AIDS Analysis Africa* 2(5): 8–9.

Kitovu. 1993. *Uganda—HIV/AIDS situation report, 1993*. Masaka: Kitovu Mobile AIDS Home Care and Orphans Programme.

———. 1994. Kitovu Mobile Home Care, Orphans and Education Programme, Annual Report, 1993. Masaka.

Kleinman A. 1978. Concepts and a model for the comparison of medical systems. *Social Science and Medicine* 12(2B): 85–93.

Koestler A. 1967. *The ghost in the machine*. London: Hutchinson.

Konde Lule J. 1995. The declining HIV seroprevalence in Uganda: What evidence? *Health Transition Review* 5(Supplement): 27–33.

Konde Lule J., S. Berkley, R. Downing. 1989. Knowledge, attitudes and practices concerning AIDS in Ugandans. *AIDS* 3(8): 513–518.

Konings E., G. Bantebya, M. Carael, D. Bagenda, T. Mertens. 1995. Validating population surveys for the measurement of HIV/STD prevention indicators. *AIDS* 9(4): 375–382.

Korenromp E., R. White, K. Orroth, R. Bakker, A. Kamali, D. Serwadda, R. Gray, H. Grosskurth, J. Habbema, R. Hayes. 2005. Determinants of the impact of sexually transmitted infection treatment on prevention of HIV infection: A synthesis of evidence from the Mwanza, Rakai, and Masaka Intervention Trials. *Journal of Infectious Diseases* 191(Supplement 1): S168–S178.

Kotler P., and G. Zaltman. 1971. Social marketing: An approach to planned social change. *Journal of Marketing* 35:3–12.

Kreiss J., D. Koech, F. Plummer, K. Holmes, M. Lightfoote, P. Piot, A. Ronald, et al. 1986. AIDS virus infection in Nairobi prostitutes. Spread of the epidemic to East Africa. *New England Journal of Medicine* 314(7): 414–418.

Kuhn T. 1962. *The structure of scientific revolutions*. Chicago: University of Chicago.

Kyaddondo D., and S. Whyte. 2003. Working in a decentralized system: A threat to health workers' respect and survival in Uganda. *International Journal of Health Planning and Management* 18(4): 329–342.

Laga M. 1995. STD control for HIV prevention—It works! *Lancet* 346(8974): 518–519.

Laga M., A. Manoka, M. Kivuvu, B. Malele, M. Tuliza, N. Nzila, J. Goeman, et al. 1993. Non-ulcerative sexually transmitted diseases as risk factors for HIV-1 transmission in women: Results from a cohort study. *AIDS* 7(1): 95–102.

Laga M., M. Alary, N. Nzila, A. Manoka, M. Tuliza, F. Behets, J. Goeman, M. St. Louis, P. Piot. 1994. Condom promotion, sexually transmitted diseases treatment, and declining incidence of HIV-1 infection in female Zairian sex workers. *Lancet* 344(8917): 246–248.

Lagerros Y. 2009. Physical activity—The more we measure, the more we know how to measure. *European Journal of Epidemiology* 24(3): 119–122.

Laing R., and C. Hodgkin. 2006. Overview of antiretroviral therapy, adherence and drug-resistance. In *From access to adherence: The challenges of antiretroviral treatment. Studies from Botswana, Tanzania and Uganda*, ed. A Hardon, 23–31. Geneva: WHO.

Lancet. 2001. Strengthening research capacity's weakest link. *Lancet* 358(9291): 1381.

Lavis J., F. Posada, A. Haines, E. Osei. 2004. Use of research to inform public policy making. *Lancet* 364(9445): 1615–1621.

Law J. 2000. On the subject of the object: Narrative, technology, and interpellation. *Configurations* 8:1–29.

Life Guard. 1997. Advertisement: *"For guys who care about what they wear."* Kampala.

Linde C. 1993. *Life stories: The creation of coherence.* New York: Oxford University Press.

Lipsitch M., and M. Nowak. 1995. The evolution of virulence in sexually transmitted HIV/AIDS. *Journal of Theoretical Biology* 174(4): 427–440.

Lipsky M. 1980. *Street-level bureaucracy: Dilemmas of the individual in public services.* New York: Russell Sage Foundation.

Low N. 2004. Review: Stephenson J, Imrie J, Bonell C. 2003. Effective sexual health interventions. Issues in experimental design. Oxford: Oxford University Press. *International Journal of Epidemiology* 33(2): 435.

Low-Beer D. 2004. Behaviour change in the HIV trials in Rakai, Masaka and Mwanza. *AIDS* 18(2): 360–361.

Lwegaba A. 1984. *Preliminary report of an "unusual wasting disease" complex nicknamed "Slim"—A slow epidemic in Rakai District, Uganda.* Report for the Ministry of Health.

Lyons. 1999. Medicine and morality: A review of responses to sexually transmitted diseases in Uganda in the twentieth century. In *Histories of sexually transmitted diseases and HIV/AIDS in sub-Saharan Africa*, ed. P. Setel et al., 97–117. Westport, CT: Greenwood Press.

Macintyre S., I. Chalmers, R. Horton, R. Smith. 2001. Using evidence to inform health policy: Case study. *British Medical Journal* 322(7280): 222–225.

Mahoney J. 2000. Path dependence in historical sociology. *Theory and Society* 29(4): 507–548.

Mandela N. 2000. Closing address, Thirteenth International AIDS Conference, Durban. http://www.anc.org.za/ancdocs/history/mandela/2000/nm0714.html. Accessed November 24, 2009.

Marseille E., P. Hofmann, J. Kahn. 2002. HIV prevention before HAART in sub-Saharan Africa. *Lancet* 359(9320): 1851–1856.

Marshall G., J. Blacklock, C. Cameron, N. Capon, R. Cruickshank, J. Gaddum, F. Heaf, et al. 1948. Streptomycin treatment of pulmonary tuberculosis. A Medical Research Council investigation. *British Medical Journal* 2(4582): 769–782.

Matteson D., J. Burr, J. Marshal. 1998. Infant mortality: A multi-level analysis of individual and community risk factors. *Social Science and Medicine* 47(11): 1841–1854.

Mbulaiteye S., C. Mahe, J. Whitworth, A. Ruberantwari, J. Nakiyingi, A. Ojwiya, A. Kamali. 2002. Declining HIV-1 incidence and associated prevalence over 10 years in a rural population in south-west Uganda: A cohort study. *Lancet* 360(9326): 41–46.

Mbulaiteye S., J. Nakiyingi, A. Ruberantwari, A. Kamali. 2000. *Falling HIV incidence: One decade of follow-up of a rural cohort in south-west Uganda.* Abstract LbPp107, Thirteenth International AIDS Conference, Durban.

McKee M. 2004. Not everything that counts can be counted; not everything that can be counted counts. *British Medical Journal* 328(7432): 153.

McQueen D. 2000. Perspectives on health promotion: Theory, evidence, practice and the emergence of complexity. *Health Promotion International* 15(2): 95–97.

———. 2002. The evidence debate. *Journal of Epidemiology and Community Health* 56:83–84.

Mexico Statement on Health Research. 2004. Knowledge for better health: Strengthening health systems. www.who.int/rpc/summit/agenda/Mexico_Statement-English.pdf. Accessed November 24, 2009.

MoH. 1989. *Progress on the AIDS epidemic in Uganda, 1987–89.* Entebbe: Ministry of Health.

———. 2000. *Health sector strategic plan 2000/1–2004/5.* Kampala: Ministry of Health.

———. 2003a. *Antiretroviral treatment policy for Uganda,* June 2003. Kampala: Ministry of Health.

———. 2003b. *National antiretroviral treatment and care guidelines for adults and children.* 1st ed., August 2003. Kampala: Ministry of Health.

———. 2005. Patient adherence to anti retroviral therapy: A situation analysis and comparison of different anti-retroviral therapy programmes in Uganda. Collaborative operations research proposal, submitted to Tropical Diseases Research Program, WHO. Kampala.

Monitor. 2001. AIDS now kills more adults than malaria. August 16. Kampala.

———. 2003. First Lady cautions on condom use. October 3. Kampala.

———. 2004. Mulago runs out of oxygen. November 10. Kampala.

———. 2005. UN attacks Uganda HIV/AIDS strategy. August 31. Kampala.

———. 2006. More than 78,000 Ugandans on ARVs, says Muhwezi. June 14. Kampala.

Morgan D., C. Mahe, B. Mayanja, J. Okongo, R. Lubega, J. Whitworth. 2002. HIV-1 infection in rural Africa: Is there a difference in median time to AIDS and survival compared with that in industrialized countries? *AIDS* 16(4): 597–603.

Moses S., F. Plummer, E. Ngugi, N. Nagelkerke, A. Anzala, J. Ndinya-Achola. 1991. Controlling HIV in Africa: Effectiveness and cost of an intervention in a high-frequency STD transmitter core group. *AIDS* 5(4): 407–411.

Moynihan R. 2004. *Using health research in policy and practice: Case studies from nine countries.* New York: Millbank Memorial Fund.

MRC. 1992. *Annual report.* Entebbe: Medical Research Council Programme on AIDS.

———. 1993. *Outlines and field protocols for a trial of IEC and IEC-STD interventions in Masaka district.* Entebbe: Medical Research Council Programme on AIDS.

MSF. 2009. *Punishing success? Early signs of a retreat from commitment to HIV/AIDS care and treatment.* Campaign for Access to Essential Medicines, Médecins Sans Frontières. Geneva.

Mugyenyi P. 2004. *ART in Uganda*. Annual conference, Uganda Medical Association. Kampala.

Muraskin W. 1996. Origins of the CVI—Intellectual foundations. *Social Science and Medicine* 42(12): 1703–1719.

Museveni Y. 1997. *Sowing the mustard seed*. London: Macmillan.

Museveni Y. 2003. United Nations or not? http://www.bbc.co.uk/radio4/news/un/transcripts/transcript_programme4.shtml. Accessed November 24, 2009.

Musumba P. 1997. Report on the policy framework for establishing program priorities to control HIV/AIDS in Uganda. Kampala: Parliamentary report.

New Vision. 1997a. Uganda: Quiet condom promotion dropped. October 29. Kampala.

———. 1997b. Cardinal Wamala maintains stand on condom. November 3. Kampala.

———. 1997c. Cheaper HIV drugs on the way. November 6. Kampala.

———. 1997d. AIDS drugs welcome. May 12. Kampala.

———. 2000a. Kazibwe disagrees with Cardinal over condoms. January 21. Kampala.

———. 2000b. Condom demand soars. February 18. Kampala.

———. 2001. AIDS centres mooted. September 10. Kampala.

———. 2002a. Condoms minor cause of HIV decline. December 16. Kampala.

———. 2002b. Janet at AIDS meet. February 26. Kampala.

———. 2003a. More patients to get HIV drugs free by 2005. August 26. Kampala.

———. 2003b. More free anti-retroviral drugs for Uganda. September 17. Kampala.

———. 2004a. Museveni condom remarks clarified. July 17. Kampala.

———. 2004b. Museveni insists condoms unsafe. October 11. Kampala.

———. 2004c. Govt. downplays condoms. November 26. Kampala.

———. 2004d. Editorial: Museveni correct on condom limits. July 16. Kampala.

New York Times. 1979. Ugandan town reported captured. February 26. New York.

———. 1980. A year after ouster of Amin, Uganda's woes continue. April 12. New York.

———. 1991. Spread of AIDS is worrying Uganda. January 30. New York.

———. 2000. South Africa in a furore over advice about AIDS. March 19. New York.

Njoroge J. 2005. AIDS fight "needs science to translate into policy." http://www.scidev.net/News/index.cfm?fuseaction=readnews&itemid=2251&language=1. Accessed November 11, 2009.

Ntozi J., and C. Kirunga. 1997. HIV/AIDS, change in sexual behaviour and community attitudes in Uganda. *Health Transition Review* 7(Supplement): 157–174.

Nutbeam D. 1999. The challenge to provide "evidence" in health promotion. *Health Promotion International* 14(2): 99–101.

O'Farrell N. 2003. Syndromic STI and behaviour-change interventions in Uganda. *Lancet* 361(9358): 2085.

O'Neil M. 2005. What determines the influence that research has on policy-making? *Journal of International Development* 17(6): 761–764.

Oakley A., D. Fullerton, J. Holland. 1995. Behavioural interventions for HIV/AIDS prevention. *AIDS* 9(5): 479–486.

Obbo C. 1995. Gender, age and class: Discourses on HIV transmission and control in Uganda. In *Culture and sexual risk: Anthropological perspectives on AIDS*, ed. H. Brummelhuis, 79–95. Amsterdam: Overseas Publishers Association.

ODI. 2004a. *Bridging research and policy on HIV/AIDS—Framework for assessing research-policy links*. London: Overseas Development Institute.

———. 2004b. *Bridging research and policy on HIV/AIDS—Workshop and project development*. London: Overseas Development Institute.

———. 2006. Theoretical models. http://www.odi.org.uk/RAPID/Tools/Theory/Index.html. Accessed, November 25, 2009.

OED. 2005. *Oxford English dictionary*. Oxford: Oxford University Press.

Offenstadt G., P. Pinta, P. Hericord, M. Jagueux, F. Jean, P. Amstutz, S. Valade, P. Lesavre. 1983. Multiple opportunistic infection due to AIDS in a previously healthy black woman from Zaire. *New England Journal of Medicine* 308(13): 775.

Okuonzi S. 2004. Dying for economic growth? Evidence of a flawed economic policy in Uganda. *Lancet* 364(9445): 1632–1637.

Opio A., V. Mishra, R. Hong, J. Musinguzi, W. Kirungi, A. Cross, J. Mermin, R. Bunnell. 2008. Trends in HIV-related behaviors and knowledge in Uganda, 1989–2005: Evidence of a shift toward more risk-taking behaviors. *Journal of Acquired Immune Deficiency Syndromes* 49(3): 320–326.

Papadopulos-Eleopulos E., V. Turner, J. Papadimitriou, B. Page, D. Causer, H. Alfonso, S. Mhlongo, T. Miller, A. Maniotis, C. Fiala. 2004. A critique of the Montagnier evidence for the HIV/AIDS hypothesis. *Medical Hypotheses* 63(4): 597–601.

Parkhurst J. 2002. The Ugandan success story? Evidence and claims of HIV-1 prevention. *Lancet* 360(9326): 78–80.

———. 2005. The response to HIV/AIDS and the construction of national legitimacy: Lessons from Uganda. *Development and Change* 36(3): 571–590.

Parkhurst J., and L. Lush. 2004. The political environment of HIV: Lessons from a comparison of Uganda and South Africa. *Social Science and Medicine* 59(9): 1913–1924.

Paterson D., S. Swindells, J. Mohr, M. Brester, E. Vergis, C. Squier, M. Wagener, N. Singh. 2000. Adherence to protease inhibitor therapy and outcomes in patients with HIV infection. *Annals of Internal Medicine* 133(1): 21–30.

PEPFAR. 2005. Implementing the ABC approach. http://www.pepfar.gov/guidance/75852.htm. Accessed November 25, 2009.

———. 2008. 2008 country profile: Uganda. http://www.pepfar.gov/documents/organization/116234.pdf. Accessed November 25, 2009.

Phair J., K. Holmes, W. Curioso, D. Heier, E. King, J. Hawes, B. Nodell. 2005. New insights into prevention of HIV and other sexually transmitted infections. Clinical care options, Northwestern University's Feinberg School of Medicine. http://faculty.washington.edu/wcurioso/holmes.pdf. Accessed November 24, 2009.

Philpott A., D. Mayer, H. Grosskurth. 2002. Translating HIV/AIDS research findings into policy: Lessons from a case study of the Mwanza trial. *Health Policy and Planning* 17(2): 196–201.

Pickering H., M. Quigley, J. Pépin, J. Todd, A. Wilkins. 1993. The effects of posttest counselling on condom use among prostitutes in The Gambia. *AIDS* 7(2): 271–273.

Piot P., J. Kreiss, J. Ndinya-Achola, E. Ngugi, J. Simonsen, D. Cameron, H. Taelman, F. Plummer. 1987. Heterosexual transmission of HIV. *AIDS* 1(4): 199–206.

Piot P., T. Quinn, H. Taelman, F. Feinsod, K. Minlangu, O. Wobin, N. Mbendi. 1984. Acquired immunodeficiency syndrome in a heterosexual population in Zaire. *Lancet* 324(8394): 65–69.

Population Reports. 1999. *Closing the condom gap.* Baltimore, MD: Johns Hopkins School of Public Health. http://info.k4health.org/pr/h9edsum.shtml. Accessed November 24, 2009.

Poulos R., and A. Zwi. 2005. Evidence-based policy making? *Medical Journal of Australia* 182(8): 429.

Powles J., and N. Day. 2003. Syndromic STI and behaviour-change interventions in Uganda. *Lancet* 361(9374): 2086.

Press I. 1990. Levels of explanation and cautions for a critical clinical anthropology. *Social Science and Medicine* 30(9): 1001–1009.

Price N., and K. Hawkins. 2002. Researching sexual and reproductive behaviour: A peer ethnographic approach. *Social Science and Medicine* 55(8): 1325–1336.

Putzel J. 2004. The politics of action on AIDS: A case study of Uganda. *Public Administration and Development* 24(1): 19–30.

Quigley M., A. Kamali, J. Kinsman, I. Kamulegeya, J. Nakiyingi-Miiro, S. Kiwuwa, J. Kengeya-Kayondo, L. Carpenter, J. Whitworth. 2004. The impact of attending a behavioural intervention on HIV incidence in Masaka, Uganda. *AIDS* 18(15): 2055–2063.

Quinn T., J. Mann, J. Curran, P. Piot. 1986. AIDS in Africa: An epidemiologic paradigm. *Science* 234(4779): 955–963.

Rakai Project. 1991. *Rakai Project: HIV dynamics and prevention, Rakai district, Uganda.* Entebbe.

Randal J. 1999. Randomized controlled trials mark a golden anniversary. *Journal of the National Cancer Institute* 91(1): 10–12.

RAWOO. 1999. Building bridges in research for development, 1997–98. RAWOO Review Report, Netherlands Development Assistance Research Council.

———. 2002. Making social science matter in the fight against HIV/AIDS. RAWOO Publication Number 24, Netherlands Development Assistance Research Council.

Richens J., J. Imrie, A. Copas. 2000. Condoms and seat belts: The parallels and the lessons. *Lancet* 355(9201): 400–403.

Robinson N., D. Mulder, B. Auvert, R. Hayes. 1997. Proportion of HIV infections attributable to other sexually transmitted diseases in a rural Ugandan population: Simulation model estimates. *International Journal of Epidemiology* 26(1): 180–189.

Rutherford G. 2002. Rapporteur session: Prevention science, Fourteenth International AIDS Conference, Barcelona. *Enfermedades Emergentes* 4(2): 82–90.

Rychetnik L., M. Frommer, P. Hawe, A. Shiell. 2002. Criteria for evaluating evidence on public health interventions. *Journal of Epidemiology and Community Health* 56(2): 119–127.

Sabatier P. 1993. Policy change over a decade or more. In *Policy change and learning: An advocacy coalition approach*, ed. P. Sabatier and H. Jenkins-Smith, 13–39. Boulder, CO: Westview Press.

Sachs J. 2001. *Macroeconomics and health: Investing in health for economic development.* Report of the Commission on Macroeconomics and Health. http://whqlibdoc.who.int/publications/2001/924154550x.pdf. Accessed November 24, 2009.

Saxinger W., P. Levine, A. Dean, G. de The, G. Lange-Wantzin, J. Moghissi, F. Laurent, M. Hoh, M. Sarngadharan, R. Gallo. 1985. Evidence for exposure to HTLV-III in Uganda before 1973. *Science* 227(4690): 1036–1038.

Schmid G. P., A. Buvé, P. Mugyenyi, G. Garnett, R. Hayes, B. Williams, J. Calleja. 2004. Transmission of HIV-1 infection in sub-Saharan Africa and effect of elimination of unsafe injections. *Lancet* 363(9407): 482–488.

Schopper D., S. Doussantousse, N. Ayiga, G. Ezatirale, W. Idro, J. Homsy. 1995. Village-based AIDS prevention in a rural district in Uganda. *Health Policy and Planning* 10(2): 171–180.

Sciortino R. 1992. Care-takers of cure: A study of health centre nurses in rural central Java. PhD Dissertation, Free University of Amsterdam.

Serwadda D., R. Mugerwa, N. Sewankambo, A. Lwegaba, J. Carswell, G. Kirya, A. Bayley, R. Downing, R. Tedder, S. Clayden. 1985. Slim disease: A new disease in Uganda, and its association with HTLV-III infection. *Lancet* 326(8460): 849–852.

Serwadda D., W. Carswell, W. Ayuko, W. Wamukota, P. Madda, R. Downing. 1986. Further experience with Kaposi's sarcoma in Uganda. *British Journal of Cancer* 53(4): 497–500.

Sewankambo N., M. Wawer, R. Gray, D. Serwadda, C. Li, R. Stallings, S. Musgrave, J. Konde-Lule. 1994. Demographic impact of HIV infection in rural Rakai district, Uganda: Results of a population-based cohort study. *AIDS* 8(12): 1707–1713.

Sewankambo N., W. Carswell, R. Mugerwa, G. Lloyd, P. Kataaha, R. Downing, S. Lucas. 1987. HIV infection through normal heterosexual contact in Uganda. *AIDS* 1(2): 113–116.

Shafer L., and A. Opio. 2006. *HIV prevalence and incidence are no longer falling in Uganda: A case for renewed prevention efforts. Evidence from a rural population cohort and from ANC surveillance.* Abstract ThLB0108, Sixteenth International AIDS Conference, Toronto.

Shelton J., D. Halperin, V. Nantulya, M. Potts, H. Gayle, K. Holmes. 2004. Partner reduction is crucial for balanced "ABC" approach to HIV prevention. *British Medical Journal* 328(7444): 891–894.

Shore C., and S. Wright. 1997. Policy: A new field of anthropology. In *Anthropology of policy: Critical perspectives on governance and power*, ed. C. Shore and S. Wright, 3–33. New York: Routledge.

Shuey D., B. Babishangire, S. Omiat, H. Bagarukayo. 1999. Increased sexual abstinence among in-school adolescents as a result of school health education in Soroti district, Uganda. *Health Education Research—Theory and Practice* 14(3): 411–419.

Silva K. 1997. "Public health" for whose benefit? Multiple discourses on malaria in Sri Lanka. *Medical Anthropology* 17(3): 195–214.

Sommerfeld J. 1994. Emerging epidemic diseases: Anthropological perspectives. *Annals of the New York Academy of Sciences* 740(1): 276–284.

Southern African Economist. 1992. Looking for a miracle. *Southern African Economist* 5(2): 5.

Star. 1984. Mysterious disease kills 100 people in Rakai. December 29. Kampala.

Stephenson J. 1999. Evaluation of behavioural interventions in HIV/STI prevention. *Sexually Transmitted Infections* 75(1): 69–71.

Stephenson J., J. Imrie, S. Sutton. 2000. Rigorous trials of sexual behaviour interventions in STD/HIV prevention: What can we learn from them? *AIDS* 14(Supplement 3): S115–S124.

Stephenson J., and F. Cowan. 2003. Evaluating interventions for HIV prevention in Africa. *Lancet* 361(9358): 633–634.

Stigler S. 1986. *The history of statistics.* Cambridge, MA: Belknap Press.

Stone L. 1986. Primary health care for whom? Village perspectives from Nepal. *Social Science and Medicine* 2(3): 293–302.

Stoneburner R., and D. Low-Beer. 2004. Population-level HIV declines and behavioral risk avoidance in Uganda. *Science* 304(5671): 714–718.

Streefland P. 1998. Epidemics and social change. In *Problems and potential in international health: Transdisciplinary perspectives,* ed. P. Streefland, 51–70. Amsterdam: Het Spinhuis.

Sunday Independent. 2000. Mbeki's AIDS call alarms scientists. March 18. Johannesburg.

Sydney Morning Herald. 1987. Condoms not answer, says African. July 21. Sydney.

Taylor J., A. Templeton, C. Vogel, J. Ziegler, S. Kyalwazi. 1971. Kaposi's sarcoma in Uganda: A clinico-pathological study. *International Journal of Cancer* 8(1): 122–135.

Tebere R. 1991. Uganda opens up new fronts. *WorldAIDS* (14): 3–4.

Terris-Prestholt F., L. Kumaranayake, S. Foster, A. Kamali, J. Kinsman, V. Basajja, N. Nalweyso, M. Quigley, J. Kengeya-Kayondo, J. Whitworth. 2006. The role of community acceptance over time for costs of HIV and STI prevention interventions: Analysis of the Masaka Intervention Trial, Uganda, 1996–1999. *Sexually Transmitted Diseases* 33(10): S111–S116.

Thorndike E., and R. Woodworth. 1901. The influence of improvement in one mental function upon the efficiency of other functions. *Psychology Review* 8:247–261, 384–395, 553–564.

Thornton R. 2008. *Unimagined community—Sex, networks, and AIDS in Uganda and South Africa.* Berkeley: University of California Press.

Tibomanya P. 1992. Kitovu-based AIDS home care service gets inspiration from orphan compassion and caring. Masaka: Kitovu Hospital report.

Tilley N., and G. Laycock. 2000. Joining up research, policy and practice about crime. *Policy Studies* 21(3): 213–227.

Times. 2003a. An ABC of AIDS—New studies give no cause to question anti-HIV treatment. February 21. London.

———. 2003b. British tests still blame sex for AIDS. February 21. London.

Tones K., and J. Green. 2004. *Health promotion—Planning and strategies*. London: Sage Publications.

UAC. 1992. Uganda AIDS Commission Statute. Kampala: Uganda AIDS Commission.

———. 1993. *HIV/AIDS national research needs assessment*. Kampala: Uganda AIDS Commission.

———. 1995. *National policy proposals on HIV/AIDS control and prevention in Uganda*. Kampala: Uganda AIDS Commission.

———. 1997. HIV Drug Access Initiative. In *National AIDS documentation and information centre bulletin*, December. Kampala: Uganda AIDS Commission.

———. 2000. *The national strategic framework for HIV/AIDS activities in Uganda: 2000/1–2005/6*. March 2000. Kampala: Uganda AIDS Commission.

———. 2002. *HIV/AIDS in Uganda: The epidemic and the response*. Kampala: Uganda AIDS Commission.

Uganda Bureau of Statistics. 2002a. Projected midyear population by region and district based on census 2002. Kampala.

———. 2002b. 2002 Uganda population and housing census, main report. Kampala.

UNAIDS. 1998. Report on the global HIV/AIDS epidemic. Geneva.

———. 2000. Report on the global HIV/AIDS epidemic. Geneva.

———. 2004. Guidelines for effective use of data from HIV surveillance systems. Geneva.

———. 2006. Report on the global AIDS epidemic: A UNAIDS 10th anniversary special edition. Geneva.

———. 2008. Report on the global AIDS epidemic. Geneva.

UNICEF. 1996. Into the 21st century: Life skills education resource booklet—Helping young Ugandans to be strong and to make choices for a bright and safe future. Kampala.

USAID. 2002. The "ABCs" of HIV prevention: Report of a USAID technical meeting on behavior change approaches to primary prevention of HIV/AIDS. http://www.usaid.gov/our_work/global_health/aids/TechAreas/prevention/abc.pdf. Accessed November 25, 2009.

Van de Perre P., D. Rouvroy, P. Lepage, J. Bogaerts, P. Kestelyn, J. Kayihigi, A. Hekker, J. Butzler, N. Clumeck. 1984. Acquired immunodeficiency syndrome in Rwanda. *Lancet* 324(8394): 62–65.

Van de Ven P., and P. Aggleton. 1999. What constitutes evidence in HIV/AIDS education? *Health Education Research—Theory and Practice* 14(4): 461–471.

Van den Borne F. 2005. *Trying to survive in times of poverty and AIDS: Women and multiple partner sex in Malawi*. Amsterdam: Het Spinhuis.

Van der Geest S. 2003. Confidentiality and pseudonyms: A fieldwork dilemma from Ghana. *Anthropology Today* 19(1): 14–18.

Van der Geest S., and A. Hardon. 2006. Social and cultural efficacies of medicines: Complications for antiretroviral therapy. *Journal of Ethnobiology and Ethnomedicine* 2:48. doi: 10.1186/1746-4269-2-48.

Van der Geest S., J. Kinsman, A. Hardon. 2010. La chaîne des médicaments en tant que phénomène multiniveau: Le cas des médicaments antirétroviraux. Notes méthodologiques et théoriques. In *Turbulences dans la chaîne des médicaments*, ed. C. Garnier and A.-L. Saives. Les éditions Liber, Montréal.

Van der Geest S., J. Speckmann, P. Streefland. 1990. Primary health care in a multi-level perspective: Towards a research agenda. *Social Science and Medicine* 30(9): 1025–1034.

Van Zyl D. 2003. *An overview of HIV-related research in Namibia since independence.* Briefing Paper No. 21. Windhoek: Institute for Public Policy Research.

Vittecoq D., and J. Modai. 1983. AIDS in a black Malian. *Lancet* 322(8357): 1023.

Wabwire-Mangen F., M. Odiit, W. Kirungi, D. Kaweesa Kisitu, J. Okara Wanyama. 2009. *Uganda: HIV modes of transmission and prevention response analysis.* Kampala: Uganda National AIDS Commission.

Wagner U., S. Malamba, G. Maude, M. Okongo, A. Kamali, J. Kengeya-Kayondo. 1992. *Muslims at lower risk of HIV-1 infection in rural SW Uganda: Circumcision or other lifestyle factors?* Abstract no. PoC 4346, Eighth International AIDS Conference, Amsterdam.

Wainberg M. 2003. *Overcoming the challenge of HIV drug resistance.* Keynote address, Fifteenth International Society for STD Research conference, Ottawa.

Walt G. 1994. *Health policy: An introduction to process and power.* London: Zed books.

Walt G., and L. Gilson. 1994. Reforming the health sector in developing countries: The central role of policy analysis. *Health Policy and Planning* 9(4): 353–370.

Walt G., L. Lush, J. Ogden. 2003. International organisations in transfer of infectious diseases policy: Iterative loops of adoption, adaptation and marketing. *Future Governance*, Paper 16.

Washington Times. 2003. Uganda leads by example on AIDS. March 13. Washington, D.C.

Wasserheit J. 1992. Epidemiological synergy. Interrelationships between human immunodeficiency virus infection and other sexually transmitted diseases. *Sexually Transmitted Diseases* 19(2): 61–77.

Wawer M., D. Serwadda, R. Gray, N. Sewankambo, C. Li, F. Nalugoda, T. Lutalo, J. Konde-Lule. 1997. Trends in HIV-1 prevalence may not reflect trends in incidence in mature epidemics: Data from the Rakai population-based cohort, Uganda. *AIDS* 11(8): 1023–1030.

Wawer M., N. Sewankambo, D. Serwadda, T. C. Quinn, L. Paxton, N. Kiwanuka, F. Wabwire-Mangen, et al. 1999. Control of sexually transmitted diseases for AIDS prevention in Uganda: A randomised community trial. *Lancet* 353(9152): 525–535.

Wawer M., R. Gray, D. Serwadda, Z. Namukwaya, F. Makumbi, N. Sewankambo, X. Li, T. Lutalo, F. Nalugoda, T. Quinn. 2005. *Declines in HIV prevalence in Uganda: Not as simple as ABC.* Abstract 27LB, Twelfth Conference on Retroviruses and Opportunistic Infections, Boston.

Wawer M., R. Gray, N. Sewankambo, D. Serwadda, L. Paxton, S. Berkley, D. McNairn, et al. 1998. A randomized, community trial of intensive sexually transmitted disease control for AIDS prevention, Rakai, Uganda. *AIDS* 12(10): 1211–1225.

Weekly Topic. 1991. Protector condom advertisement, August 23. Kampala.

Weeks D. 1992. The AIDS pandemic in Africa. *Current History* 91(565): 208–213.

Weidle P., S. Malamba, R. Mwebaze, C. Sozi, G. Rukundo, R. Downing, D. Hanson, et al. 2002. Assessment of a pilot antiretroviral drug therapy programme in Uganda: Patients' response, survival, and drug resistance. *Lancet* 360(9326): 34–40.

White R., K. Orroth, E. Korenromp, R. Bakker, M. Wambura, N. Sewankambo, R. Gray, et al. 2004. Can population differences explain the contrasting results of the Mwanza, Rakai, and Masaka HIV/sexually transmitted disease intervention trials? A modelling study. *Journal of AIDS* 37(4): 1500–1513.

WHO. 1977. Smallpox surveillance. *Weekly Epidemiological Record* 52(49): 389–391.

———. 1978. *Declaration of Alma-Ata International Conference on Primary Health Care, Alma-Ata, USSR, 6–12 September 1978.* www.who.int/hpr/NPH/docs/declaration_almaata.pdf. Accessed November 21, 2009.

———. 1991. *Management of patients with sexually transmitted diseases.* World Health Organisation Technical Report Series, Number 810. Geneva.

———. 1998. Resolution of the Executive Board of the WHO on health promotion. *Health Promotion International* 13(3): 266.

———. 2002a. Fourteenth World AIDS Conference: International Collaboration in Scaling Up the Response to AIDS. http://www.who.int/director-general/speeches/2002/english/20020709_InternationalCollaborationScalingUptheRResponsetoAIDS.html. Accessed November 25, 2009.

———. 2002b. *Scaling up antiretroviral therapy in resource-limited settings: Guidelines for a public health approach.* http://www.who.int/hiv/pub/prev_care/en/ScalingUp_E.pdf. Accessed December 12, 2009.

———. 2006a. *Important progress seen in tackling AIDS, but epidemic continues to outpace response, says new comprehensive global AIDS update.* http://www.who.int/hiv/mediacentre/news60/en/index.html. Accessed November 25, 2009.

———. 2006b. *The '3 by 5' initiative.* http://www.who.int/3by5/en/. Accessed November 25, 2009.

———. 2006c. *Evidence to improve HIV treatment and prevention programmes: Operational research to support HIV treatment and prevention in resource-limited settings. Summary of Activities, July 2004 to January 2006.* Geneva.

———. 2009a. *Towards universal access—Scaling up priority HIV/AIDS interventions in the health sector. Progress Report 2009.* Geneva. http://www.who.int/hiv/pub/2009progressreport/en/index.html. Accessed December 9, 2009.

————. 2009b. *Rapid advice—Antiretroviral therapy for HIV infection in adults and adolescents*. http://www.who.int/hiv/pub/arv/rapid_advice_art.pdf. Accessed December 12, 2009.

WHO/UNAIDS. 2003. *Treating 3 million by 2005—Making it happen*. http://www.who.int/3by5/publications/documents/en/3by5StrategyMakingItHappen.pdf. Accessed November 25, 2009.

Whyte S. 1992. Pharmaceuticals as folk medicine: Transformations in the social relations of health care in Uganda. *Culture, Medicine and Psychiatry* 16(2): 163–186.

Whyte S., M. Whyte, L. Meinert, D. Kyaddondo. 2003. Treating AIDS: Dilemmas of unequal access in Uganda. In *Global pharmaceuticals: Ethics, markets, practices*, ed. A. Petryna, A. Kleinman, A. Lakoff, 240–262. Berkeley: University of California Press.

Wilson D. 1989. African contributions on AIDS/HIV. *AIDS Care* 1(2): 195–198.

————. 2004. Partner reduction and the prevention of HIV/AIDS. *British Medical Journal* 328(7444): 848–849.

Wilson D., and S. Lavelle. 1990. HIV/AIDS in Africa. *AIDS Care* 2(4): 371–375.

World Bank. 1993. *World development report—Investing in health*. Oxford: Oxford University Press.

————. 2003. Sexually Transmitted Infections Project. Implementation completion and results report. http://web.worldbank.org/external/projects/main?pagePK=64283627&piPK=73230&theSitePK=40941&menuPK=228424&contentFed=yes&Projectid=P002963. Accessed November 25, 2009.

WorldAIDS. 1991. *"Act now," warns Africa report*. London, September.

Yanow D. 1993. The communication of policy meanings: Implementation as interpretation and text. *Policy Sciences* 26(1): 41–61.

Youssef H. 1993. The history of the condom. *Journal of the Royal Society of Medicine* 86(4): 226–228.

Index